Unspeakable

The Things
We Cannot Say

Harriet Shawcross

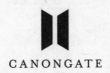

CANONGATE

This paperback edition published in 2020 by Canongate Books

First published in Great Britain, the USA and Canada in 2019
by Canongate Books Ltd, 14 High Street, Edinburgh EH1 1TE

canongate.co.uk

Distributed in the USA by Publishers Group West
and in Canada by Publishers Group Canada

1

For permissions credits please see p. 333

British Library Cataloguing-in-Publication Data
A catalogue record for this book is available on
request from the British Library

ISBN 978 1 78689 007 8

Typeset in Goudy Old Style by
Palimpsest Book Production Ltd, Falkirk, Stirlingshire

Printed and bound in Great Britain by Clays Ltd, Elcograf S.p.A.

Unspeakable

Harriet Shawcross is an award-winning filmmaker and journalist. She obtained an MA in Creative Non-Fiction from the University of East Anglia, and was shortlisted for the Manchester Fiction Prize. *Unspeakable* is her first book.

For Christa,
who always listened

How shall we say how this happened, these stories, our stories

'Anniversary Poem' by George Oppen

CONTENTS

Part Four: Silence

Part Five: Last Word

INTRODUCTION: A HANDFUL OF TEETH

ONE SUNDAY AFTERNOON I COME to sit with the dead. The room is almost untouched. Smiling graduation photos of my siblings stare back at me from the bookcase, and a Kermit the Frog with wire legs straddles the cut-glass decanter. Everything and nothing is the same. I am standing in my grandmother's study. She lived with us for twenty-five years, and died six months ago. Her room has now been cleaned and closed, the dark beetles of dried blood scrubbed from the fireplace where she fell and cracked her head, half a year before the stroke that killed her. Unusually the house is empty, and I have come to her room to sit with the silence.

I walk to the bookshelves, and run my fingers against her things, feeling the edges of her life. I lift the lid of a china sweetie jar to find a few dried-out Liquorice Allsorts. There are so many books. Dictionaries of quotations and guides to etiquette. Cordon bleu courses from the 1970s, with handwritten table plans folded between the pages. Many of the books are unmarked, simply bound in leather, gilt-edged. I pull one down from the shelf and have to laugh. It isn't a book at all. It is a VHS case, disguised as a leather-bound bible. And as I look I realise that there are dozens of these faux leather books, presumably hiding covert recordings of *Midsomer Murders* and *Foyle's War*. I crack open one of the cases, but the handwriting on the label is indecipherable, its story lost to the world. As I move along the bookshelf I remove a biography of Churchill, only to find dozens of paperback romance novels hidden behind it. It is so typical of my grandmother, who fervently believed in the power of appearance, in everything being just so. She was always immaculately turned out, and told me when I turned fifteen that I needed to start moisturising my neck every day. She slept on a silk pillow until the day she died, because she believed it was good for the skin.

Beside the biographies is a cluster of little porcelain boxes, with gold hinges. They are collectors' items, commissioned to mark important events, from the birth of a grandchild to a trip to a Broadway premiere. I lift one up, and it rattles like a sand dollar. I prise it open, struggling with the stiff gold hinges, and stop for a second. Inside are half a dozen milk teeth, yellowed pips of enamel saved from the tooth fairy's visits to my siblings, over twenty years ago. I can't believe she has kept them: this eternal marker of identity. The thing that survives when everything else is gone. Dental records – or a clattering cipher of love.

My grandmother moved in with us when I was a child. Or at the edge of being a child: thirteen. The move shifted the family dynamic. It was a time of great upheaval and change, and it was during this time that I lost the ability to speak. Or not to speak, precisely, but to speak in the ways that make us human. The ways that matter. The ways that define who we are. I could answer direct questions. I could take part in school plays. But I stopped making conversation for nearly a year. When I was at school, I stopped telling jokes, or asking questions. I became a lurker. Always almost invisible, on the edge of conversations. I would watch days pass without saying anything of substance. And I was unable to tell anyone what was happening. When my grandmother moved in with us there was a corrosion – of privacy, space and time, which meant that not everything was said. And so the new shape of the family was somehow tied to my silence.

In many ways, that year shaped the person I was to become – adept at disappearing, at watching, listening. Living off other people's lives. I have worked for the past ten years as a journalist, and I can't count the number of times I have said, 'Pretend I'm not here. Talk to the camera. Don't look at me.' The art of the interview is in disappearing – not interrupting, or filling the silences – so that the interviewee will reveal themselves. And when I wasn't working, I spent my free time volunteering for Samaritans; listening to other people's stories, as I didn't quite know how to voice my own. I have always found it hard to say how I feel, and this silence has driven my relationships to the edge of existence as I often couldn't find the words to articulate my doubts and fears, or even say I love you.

The time I stopped talking has always seemed to me to be at the absolute core of who I am. But writing about that time, when I slipped into silence for a few months, feels wrong somehow, like rooting around in my grandmother's room: moving aside the carefully constructed veneer, the metaphorical biographies, and leather-bound cassette tapes, to reveal a handful of teeth. It was a time when my parents were stretched to breaking point, bent out of shape, with compromise and worry. And I don't want to remind anyone of that, or suggest they did anything wrong. Because behind it all was love: a clutch of baby teeth in boxes. It was only ever love.

Now my grandmother has gone, the family is resetting, taking new shape like a broken bone. We are learning to rebalance the weight. My parents are selling the house. They are moving away. Starting again. And I am getting married.

It is strange living in this hiatus before everything changes, and I become somebody's wife. In some ways it feels that in getting married I am finally standing up and taking hold of language to change something in the physical world – I do. And perhaps that is why I have found my mind turning to those first silent years. It feels important to understand why I stopped speaking, in a way that it never has before. And so for the first time I have started trying to think my way back into those empty days, revisiting memories that have lain dormant for years. And I have begun tentatively reaching out to others to try and find out how they coped when words failed them. I hope that by understanding how language can desert other people, I may get to the heart of what happened to me – so that I can exorcise silence from my life, once and for all.

I have come to my grandmother's room to try and find

something to read at the wedding. She always taught me poetry was important – and that you needed other people's words to fall back on when your own fail. Her legacy to me was a small white suitcase filled with poetry that she had torn out of books and magazines or copied out of other people's books throughout her life. But today I am stuck. The traditional poets have let me down. The internet searches for 'wedding poems' have left me with grandiloquence and metaphor that takes me further and further from how I actually feel. On website after website I read the same passages from Elizabeth Barrett Browning and Margery Williams' *The Velveteen Rabbit* about how love makes us real. The words are not working.

Marriage feels alien to me. I have been to so many weddings, but I have no sense of what it means to be married. It reminds me of a story I once read about the 'most photographed barn in America'. Everyone knew what it was, and would travel for miles to take a picture. But it was so well known, so well photographed and signposted, that no one could actually see it for what it was. It had become a simulacrum, an imitation of itself. Marriage feels a bit like that to me. Celebrated, and universally talked about – but totally unknowable. The reality of being married is strangely untethered from the word.

I scan the shelves aimlessly, picking open old copies of Rupert Brooke, and anthologies of twentieth-century love poetry. None of it is quite right. And then I see it – an old book of mine – wedged between the biographies. The spine is bound in what looks like faded green calico. I pull the book open. The pages are annotated with pencil and dog-eared. An old ticket for the

BART – the train running between San Francisco and the Bay area – is wedged between the pages.

This is George Oppen, a little-known poet of the American West and East coasts. He prided himself on saying it as it was, on stripping everything back so that language could get as close as possible to the world. But at the same time his writing is incredibly sparse. It is almost as if he doesn't want words to get in the way of the thing he is describing. The poems sit like little insects on the pages: dots against the endless white.

I first discovered Oppen when I was studying in California. I fell in love with his simplicity. I had been raised on a diet of T. S. Eliot and high Modernism. Oppen was different. He loved the little words, and seemed to have a childlike delight in the fact that the world existed, and that he could bear witness to it. I don't remember lending my book of Oppen to my grand-mother – but books would find their way into her room, from my bedroom across the hall, from time to time. I can't blame her for wandering into my room during the empty days, when she would shuffle from one end of the house to the other, ferrying the *Daily Mail* in the basket of her walker. Waiting for my parents to come home, so she would have someone to talk to.

Subconsciously I sit in the chair I would have sat in to make conversation with her. I can almost see her on the sofa. The hair that stayed red into her nineties, and that night's viewing ringed in the *Radio Times* on the table. The pillows newly plumped. This is where we would sit when we came to talk to her – often saying very little, just listening to the litany of her days.

I begin to read, and my eye is drawn to one of the shorter

poems, 'The Hills'. It was written about the poet's wife Mary – who he was married to his entire life.

> That this is I,
> Not mine, which wakes
> To where the present
> Sun pours in the present moment, to the air perhaps
> Of love and of
> Conviction.

I pause. I think I have found it. This moment of bright optimism – of not knowing what would happen next – is exactly how I feel. And wanting to hold onto each other without taking ownership: 'I, not mine'. These are the words I want to say. This is the delicate hope of love – of knowing that now we have chosen each other, things would be different.

I close the book, and take Oppen back into my life. Perhaps he can help me – for before his words can be said at the wedding, I know I must go back into the silence. To try and understand the emptiness that stalked my early schooldays and seeped into the most intimate corners of my life, bending relationships out of shape and driving me towards work rather than intimacy. Maybe Oppen, the poet of the gaps and caesuras of gaping white space – but above all heartfelt honesty – can help me to find the words.

PART ONE

FEAR

BERKELEY

I was staying in one of the largest student cooperatives in North America, as an exchange student, when I first discovered Oppen. It was a large wooden house in the Berkeley Hills, where the air smelt of eucalyptus and weed. Students performed the building maintenance, cooking and cleaning in exchange for subsidised rent – and unbeknown to me, it was famous across campus as a party house. They once held a rave where they gave out Ecstasy tablets from a biscuit tin at the door, and spent canisters of nitrous oxide, or laughing gas, routinely littered the basketball court. Students rose on Ritalin, to steady their minds for midterms, and then sank down with weed for the weekend. The house was renovated, and refocused around academic endeavour a few years after I left, after a student died of an overdose.

The fact the house was maintained by the residents meant it always felt dark – light bulbs weren't changed and the windows rarely cleaned. The walls were covered with murals: a cow's face eyed you in the main hall, and my room was adorned with a huge wave, the nauseous swell rising above my head.

I didn't feel at home in Berkeley. And yet I never said anything. I never tried to change accommodation, or tell anyone that things weren't right. The cooperative was arranged around a courtyard, peppered with broken bottles. After a party the residents would throw the empty bottles at the wall, and I would lie in bed, listening to the glass breaking on the basketball court below. This was the year that The Facebook arrived in Berkeley and I spent hours looking at the online profiles of students in neighbouring rooms. I was out of place: I didn't get high, and I mislabelled the universe, calling cilantro 'coriander', and Band-Aids 'plasters'.

It was a time when nothing worked. Language, in particular, was broken. I remember trying to explain the peculiarly British idea that you 'can't be bothered' to write an essay to my roommate, one evening.

'Do you mean you don't want to?' she said.

'No, I *want* to, I just can't be bothered,' I replied.

'So you *can't* do it?'

'No, it's not that I can't do it. I *can* do it, and I *want* to do it – I just can't be bothered.'

But my words didn't mean anything. In a world where your parents have been saving for college since before you were born, and where undergrad is just the first rung on a decade of Grad School, Law School, Med School, Any School to prepare you for the world – the idea of not being 'bothered' with work was anathema. Even the drug-taking often seemed to me to be pushed to the level of absurdity: there was no such thing as a quiet pint on a Tuesday. You were sleeping in the library during the week, and then getting out of your mind at the weekend. I remember the first time I saw someone balling a sleeping bag into their rucksack in the stacks of the central library, I laughed. I couldn't imagine living at that level of intensity. And yet the covert sleeping bag somehow made sense of the speed, ketamine, cocaine. That was the pattern of life.

Into this came Oppen. I was lonely, and frustrated. Something about his brilliant, bright directness made sense to me. He was not trying to be clever – just saying things as they were. I was introduced to him as part of a course on Objectivist poetry. His philosophy was that poetry should always be 'sincere', and that the poem is a reflection that 'there is a moment, an actual time, when you believe something to be true'.[1] The word 'objectivist' refers to the fact that the poets saw the poem itself as an object, or artefact, which helped to explain and bear witness to real things in the world.[2] His work was taught alongside the abstruse and difficult poetry of Louis Zukofsky – and Oppen was a breath of fresh air. One of the first poems I read was about deer. It is called 'Psalm', and begins:

> In the small beauty of the forest
> The wild deer bedding down –
> That they are there![3]

As I read I could see the deer in the beech woods by the house I grew up in. The little muntjac who would dart out of sight, with a rustle of leaves, so that there was a sense of the miraculous, on the rare occasions that one stopped in your path. I understood his reverence for the world. But more than that the poem seemed to speak of a respect for language too. In the final stanza Oppen turns from the deer to the words themselves; 'The small nouns / Crying faith'.

In interviews and essays he would return to this poem, and explain that in this final verse he was simply saying that language mattered, because it referred to something real in the world. He was in awe not only of the deer, but of the words themselves, the 'small nouns' that pointed to the objects in the world and made them real: the 'wild deer' with their 'alien small teeth'.[4]

In my homesick funk, I had almost lost sight of this reverence for both the world and words. I was falling out of sync with life around me – failing to make friends and building my days around late-night Skype calls back to the UK. And so I began to hold onto Oppen in this parallel universe where language didn't work, and I couldn't connect with people. I held onto his faith in humanity. His most famous poem is called 'Of Being Numerous'. It was part of a collection that won the Pulitzer Prize in 1968. In it he seems to be trying to reconcile the paradox of being at once part of humanity and existentially alone:

Obsessed, bewildered

By the shipwreck
Of the singular

We have chosen the meaning
Of being numerous.[5]

The poem is full of images of the push and pull of isolation and community. It is packed with images of urban living, with people crushed cheek by jowl, 'Pressed, pressed on each other'. And yet, it also depicts a city of missed connections, of thresholds, doorways, 'a world of stoops', of walls and windows – the things that come between us. But the poet is not isolated, or cut off from other people by the city. Rather, he is bound by human connections that run to the bone – the ties you wish you could break, for he says:

> I cannot even now
> Altogether disengage myself
> From those men[6]

The paradox of being both desperately alone in the middle of the city, and also unable to shake the voices of others, made sense to me. It resonated with those days of glancing at the still-new Facebook, and the loneliness of cooperative living – where memories of home were more real than my neighbours' faces. The only other place I have really experienced that kind of loneliness was during my first few years of boarding school. It was a place where you were always watched, but rarely seen. I remember waking up and locking eyes with another girl across the dormitory, and the strange sadness of entering each other's consciousness before we were quite awake.

*

Back in London, after choosing the wedding poem at my parents' house, I continue to read Oppen, carrying my book of poetry on the Tube in and out of work, the small lines juddering with the motion of the train. The early poems are prefaced by Ezra Pound, the father of Modernism. Oppen was, he said, a bright young thing, a 'serious craftsman', with a 'sensibility that has not been got out of any other man's books'.[7] The first poems, gathered together in a collection called *Discrete Series*, are unmistakably of New York. Even underground in London I can feel myself there: the dark buildings that reach to the sky and the wind tunnel streets. And the wide ocean. Oppen had sailed into New York on a cat boat with his new wife Mary. I imagine him, dark and saturnine, observing the city in glances, first a 'Closed car – closed in glass – / At the curb, / Unapplied and empty'[8] and then the city ladies, 'Your coats wrapped, / Your hips a possession'.[9] He mocks the pointless spunk of capitalism, the 'prudery / of frigidaire, of / Soda-jerking –'.[10] And he seems somehow invisible, detached from the city. He is able to assess, to judge – to take a lover and see only her component parts, 'your armpits causeways for water'.[11] There is something of the journalist in these early poems, a certain distance. A certain self-assurance.

And then it stops. There is a gap. I turn the pages back and forward to try and confirm it. The next poems in my collection are from 1962. There is nothing between 1934 and 1962. Not a word for this span of a life. He has vanished. I can't understand what happened. The pictures alongside the poems also jump from a young man looking out at the sea to a seemingly ageless, wizened face, lost in the middle distance. Where has he gone? Why would he have stopped writing? I get off the Tube, flustered for a moment in the melee above ground. There must be a reasonable explanation – perhaps in his letters or personal papers there will be clues.

So I renew my membership of the British Library, and go in search of books I have not read for ten years. I wrote my university dissertation on George Oppen when I came back from America, and spent days scanning obscure journals in the silence of the Reading Rooms. But I had forgotten about this gap. It is strange that I would have forgotten that he stopped writing for almost thirty years – but then that's the thing about silence, it is at root, an absence and, in a sense, there is nothing to remember. The books are sent up from the subterranean stacks, and I open them eagerly, hoping for clues. But there is nothing. Less than nothing. It was not just his poetry that stopped. His selected letters start and then abruptly stop in the early 1930s, only to start again in 1958.[12] He kept a living correspondence throughout his life – writing several letters a day, which read like conversations. But not in those years. There is nothing. I check the archive records for the University of San Diego where Oppen's archive is stored. Alongside the letters are notes, jottings and daybooks, the notebooks in which he wrote his poetry. But again, there is nothing. The earliest letters and notes in the archive seem to date from 1957. I have hit a silence.

I feel cheated, angry almost. I want to understand why he stopped. I look around the library at the other people, heads bowed in the glow of their desk lamps, set apart like an Edward Hopper painting. They don't care. My frustration deepens when I learn from the Preface to Oppen's selected letters that while his words may have stopped, his life continued apace. He went to war, fighting the advance of Hitler during the 1940s, and then returned, wounded, to America, only to fall under the suspicion of Joseph McCarthy. In the Cold War, Oppen and his young family were seen as being suspect because of their Communist Party membership in the 1930s. And so, I learn, he went to Mexico, and lived as an exile for almost a decade, with his wife and daughter, before returning to the States in 1958.[13] But for all of this, there are no words. Just a thumbnail biographical sketch. Or at least, there are no words written at the time. It is only in the poetry and letters written in the later years of his life that Oppen begins to pick through everything that happened, sifting through and making sense of it all.

Why would a poet stop writing at the height of his career? He had been hailed as a new and distinctive voice by Ezra Pound, after all. Why would he stop taking notes, or writing letters – or at least make sure those words, if they existed, would never see the light of day? After Oppen started writing again, in the late 1950s, everything was saved – his archive contains shopping lists, fragments, endless letters, the poems carved out of the ephemera of life, as if making up for lost time. Or lost words.

Had he chosen his silence, or were there things in life he simply could not write about? Perhaps the experience of war, hinted at in 'Of Being Numerous'? Or life as an exile? It feels urgent, important – I need to know. When I chose the Oppen poem to read at the wedding I had forgotten that his life was shaped around a silence. And now it seems too great a coincidence to ignore, as I explore the pauses in my own life.

I get up and walk out of the Reading Rooms, and through the café to the verandah, which looks out across the roar of the Euston Road. Around me everyone is eating lunch. Tables of academics and students are talking on their phones and chatting. Laughing and sharing sandwiches in the sun. Listening to the drift and swell of their conversation, it feels like being underwater. It makes sense that in shaking off my own silence I would turn again to Oppen: a poet with silence at the heart of his working life – but who has somehow always found the words I have wanted to say.

THE VOLVO

My silence began in the Volvo. It was my father's car, with a towel for the dog draped across the back seat and forgotten Yorkie wrappers in the footwell.

I couldn't tell you the day I stopped talking. But I can place it, point to it, feel my way into it almost. And for me it was the Volvo, driving through the half-light of winter mornings. The flash and flare of headlights, and the dead space of the commute.

I remember being told once that during the Iranian revolution cars became figured as a space beyond politics, somewhere no one could see what was happening – safe from the secret police, immune from surveillance, where you could kiss, or talk, without being heard. Somewhere anything could happen. The Volvo felt a bit like that.

To us as children it was a tank: indestructible. My father always joked that it was special because it would always come off better than the other guy in a crash, and as a child it would take all my weight to turn the handles that lowered the windows.

It was a space for play: for reverse seats in the 'very back' that faced the receding traffic; the smell of chlorine after Sunday afternoon swimming; and sugared fingertips from sticky buns.

But all that changed when I started secondary school. The day began with an hour's commute, and the Volvo became functional: a taxi, where nothing is communicated but pleasantries.

When I started school, my father re-routed his life, and would drive an hour cross-country every morning so that he could drop me at the gates, before catching the 7.30 train into London.

We would eat breakfast together in the numb dark before dawn, and drive along the motorway listening to 'Classic Gold' on medium wave radio: 'Nights in White Satin' and 'Unchained Melody'. We rarely spoke on the journey; each staring blankly into the middle distance, as he hummed tunes from before I was born. He smelt of aftershave, and kept an electric razor in the glove box.

Ten minutes before we arrived, our route took us down a slip road, which ran alongside the motorway. My father would invariably say it was a shortcut, but I'm not sure if it saved us any time. It was my favourite part of the journey. Mist rose above football fields, and the empty goalposts stood matchstick-precarious. For a minute it felt as though we could be going anywhere. And then the black and white chevrons of a sharp turn would flash past the window, and we were back on the motorway, and the headlights of traffic crawling towards the roundabout at the top of the hill.

I often think I could have said something to my father on

that slip road – in that moment when things could be different. But I never quite found the words.

When we arrived, he would shave as we waited in the car park – stretching his skin in the rearview mirror.

'Have a good day,' he would say with a smile. 'Work hard and earn lots of money.'

In the evenings I collapsed wordlessly into the passenger seat; a strange mirror image of him, in my school shirt and tie.

'How was work?' I would ask.

'Fine. School?'

'Fine.'

'That's good.'

But things were far from good at school. I had always been popular at the village primary I had attended until I was ten years old – but in this prestigious all-girls boarding school I was lost; unmoored somehow, and set adrift. I was one of only three day-girls in a year of almost one hundred. From the start I felt like an outsider, and I had been warned not to talk about life at home.

'Now then,' the housemistress had said, at the beginning of term, 'I think it's best if you don't mention your parents too much – and try not to make a fuss when you're being picked up this evening.'

I nodded. She straightened her skirt to hide the pale hem of her petticoat.

'This is the first time most of the boarders will have been away,' she said, 'and some might get a bit homesick-y. We want you to feel welcome, of course – but we haven't had any day-girls before.' She paused. 'So this will be a learning curve for all of us.'

For the first two weeks of term the boarders were not permitted to call home. Instead, they wrote letters to their parents in Chelsea, and arrived in chapel red-eyed every morning. After this hiatus, they were allowed ten minutes, each week, to use the public payphone in the corridor.

Going home became a guilty secret. I never announced when I was leaving, but slipped silently into the junior library to wait for my father to arrive. Sitting there alone I would listen to the sing-song of the other girls' conversation, as they walked back to the boarding houses in the dark.

I struggled to fit in, and by the second year I knew something had to change. So I began to join the boarders in the dining room as they ate breakfast, in an effort to make friends. Buoyant with the morning's letters, or tearful – linking arms in solidarity – they talked of the moments I had missed overnight. Initially I tried to take part, laughing at everyone else's jokes and hovering beside fast-forming circles of friends – but without the shared reference points of dormitory life I couldn't carve a way into the conversation, and soon I began avoiding the other girls altogether.

I began to hide in the boot room during breakfast. Rows of metal cages and heavy cloaks – used only once a year for the carol service – made it an easy place to disappear. Trunks and tuck boxes were stacked to the ceiling and the air smelt of sweat and linseed oil. No one was ever there for more than a few minutes – to collect a lacrosse stick or a textbook.

'Oh, hi,' they would say, 'I didn't see you there.'

'Yeah, sorry, I was just leaving,' I'd reply.

'Cool.'

No one guessed I had been standing there for an hour, pretending to have just arrived. My days were bookended by awkward pauses in the boot room, and as time went on the silence began to swell, until I found I had nothing to say.

I never intended to stop talking – but soon keeping quiet became a habit. I felt the silence settling on me in the Volvo, as we drove down the hill towards the gates. It felt safer, easier somehow, to say the bare minimum. I would answer direct questions from teachers or other girls, but I lost the art of conversation. Looking back I find it hard to pinpoint exactly when my silence took hold in those first few years of secondary school, or to know how long it lasted. What is imprinted on my memory are individual moments. The unallocated pauses between classes, when the other girls would be saving seats, and drawing biro tattoos on the backs of their hands, as I looked on. I knew my behaviour was odd – and would try and will myself to speak – but I didn't know how to break into their conversations. Weeks would pass when I said little more than, 'Yeah. Cool. Thanks.' I was never bullied – just ignored.

My parents didn't realise what was happening. I didn't know how to tell my father on the long drive home that I had barely said a word since we had parted that morning. And once I was back in the familiar surroundings of home, I found I could talk normally again. I was ashamed of my silence – and feared I must have done something terribly wrong, if no one wanted to talk to me.

It is now more than two decades since I stopped talking at school – but silence has become a fault line running through my life – always splitting at the same points of weakness. I see my teenage self in the anxiety I still feel before parties, and the blank fear of being cornered with nothing to say. Or in memories of sitting in a university interview, as they waited for me to answer a question about the role of the gravediggers in *Hamlet,* and knowing no words would come out of my mouth. Looking back, I realise that even as a very young child I would retreat into silence when things went wrong. Even though I was popular in primary school, there were breaktimes I remember slowly walking around the edge of the netball court, treading the painted perimeter like a tightrope, when no one would play with me.

And as an adult, silence has served me well professionally. On the eve of my first filming trip to Afghanistan, for example, I was sent on a 'hostile environment course', to learn what to do if I were to be kidnapped. We were told the best way to survive was to become the metaphorical grey man in the room – the person no one would notice. Answer questions if they are asked, we were told, and try to blend in. Don't make sudden movements. Never say more than you need to.

This survival strategy was reassuringly familiar, as I had spent my early adolescence as the 'grey man' – becoming ever more quiet, unobtrusive and almost invisible at school. For me, that was the purpose of not speaking – it was a way of staying safe.

But now I realise that silence is unsustainable; it may keep the hostage alive for a few extra hours, but it is no way to build a life. Over time it has threatened everything I care about, and now I must find my way out of it.

A SPECTRE IN EVERY STREET

WHEN OPPEN RETURNED TO NEW YORK in 1933, after a brief sojourn living and working in France, he couldn't believe what he saw.[14] Fifteen million families were faced with the threat of imminent starvation, and as soon as he stepped outside, he encountered men on the streets with nothing to eat.[15] The cosmopolitan city 'walled in glass' that he had written about in *Discrete Series* had changed. The smart boutiques and confident 'city ladies' were no more. Manhattan was in the grip of the Great Depression. By 1934 twenty million people were unemployed,[16] and suddenly the self-assured young poet was at a loss. How could he write when all around him families were struggling to survive, and men were standing in breadlines?

These were real, ethical questions for Oppen. He felt deeply that he could not – should not – be writing poetry while the people around him were struggling to get by. In his one published essay on the purpose of poetry, 'The Mind's Own Place', written long after the Great Depression, he recalls the words of the dramatist Bertolt Brecht, who believed that there were times when 'it can be almost a crime to write of trees'. There are, Oppen argued, situations 'that cannot honourably be met by art'.[17] This was one of those times. Poetry was not an appropriate response to starvation.

I imagine Oppen walking through Manhattan, past breadlines three men deep, horrified by what he would later describe as a 'spectre in every street'.[18] This was not a distant, remote catastrophe – and it affected him deeply. Oppen's response to the suffering he saw around him would be played out again and again in his later poetry, as he tried to determine both who he was and what it meant to be part of society. I see this struggle in the opening lines of 'Of Being Numerous' when the poet wonders how we should relate to each other, for:

> There are things
> We live among 'and to see them
> Is to know ourselves'.[19]

The men were not remote and distant 'others' to Oppen, they were both a reflection of himself, and part of his community – 'ourselves'. They were all part of the same struggle, the same vast numerous humanity. [20]

I am shocked when I look back through the black and white images of the Depression. The faceless masses waiting outside soup kitchens in Manhattan, all still wearing their office trench coats and hats. The wooden lean-tos in the slums, with men gathered around a makeshift 'cook house', which was little more than a pan above a pile of burning garbage. I stop on one image of Christmas in Manhattan in 1931.[21] The image shows men queuing for Christmas dinner at a municipal lodging house. The line is four men deep and winds across the frame and away into the distance. There must be hundreds standing there. The cars sit empty at the kerb. For the first time I have a sense of how cataclysmic it must have been for Oppen. He had recently returned from travelling in France with Mary, living off his inheritance, as they tried to set up a publishing house. His life had been relatively care-free – and now he was face to face with starvation. He could not avoid it or walk past it; it blocked the street in endless lines leading to the steaming soup kitchens.

Both he and Mary felt they needed to do something concrete to help. Words would not do. Faced with the breadlines, Oppen believed that the 'business of everyone' was to 'come to the aid of the unemployed',[22] and so, as Mary recalls in her autobiography, the young couple said to each other, 'Let's work with the unemployed and leave our interest in the arts for a later time.'[23] And so Oppen laid aside poetry, as a way of making space for practical action.

The Oppens joined the Communist Party in 1935, and became members of the Workers Alliance, in the hope of doing something practical to improve the welfare of ordinary New Yorkers.[24] As Oppen recalled years later, 'We were interested in rioting' and 'disorder, disorder – to make it impossible to allow people to starve'.[25] Oppen became Kings County election campaign manager for the 1936 elections,[26] and the couple helped the Farmers' Union organise a milk strike in Utica, Oneida County, New York. Many of these milk strikes ended in violence, and I imagine him astride one of the milk carts, throwing the pails over his head to the street below, the milk flowing across the dirt, so that it stayed out of the hands of the state troopers, who were often sent to break up the strikes.

Once he had joined the Communist Party, Oppen didn't want to mention the fact that he was a writer. If he was known to be a poet then there was a danger that anything he wrote about his experiences of the Depression could be co-opted by the party, and used as propaganda.[27] This was a time when words were not your own; they could be twisted and turned to political ends. In later years, Oppen would explain this decision as an act of 'conscience',[28] for 'when the crisis occurred, we knew we didn't know what the world was, and we had to find out'.[29]

But his silence was not simply a bewildered retreat. There was a power in choosing not to speak. In refusing to let your words be used in the service of a political cause. I think, even as a child, I intuited that silence could be powerful; you couldn't be hurt or misunderstood if you didn't offer anything of yourself. If nothing else, silence could offer a form of protection. I admire his decision not to write, to lay poetry aside and do something practical. There have been many times as a journalist when I have wondered if it was right to keep the camera rolling, or to write scripts to summarise the suffering of others – rather than actually helping. I remember filming desperate poverty in Kabul one winter and driving backwards and forwards trying to get the right shot of a homeless woman huddled in a burka in the snow. Shouldn't we have stopped the car? It seems to me that Oppen was right; there is something ethically questionable about documenting the suffering of others for your own ends, whether that is in poetry or on film. Of course there is a value in telling and raising awareness – but somehow my sympathies lie with Oppen and Brecht, and the times when it can be a crime to speak of trees.

And yet, I think there's more to his silence. Yes, there was the ethical imperative to offer practical support rather than empty words, and also his desire to keep his work away from the propaganda machine, but there seems to be a third strand to Oppen's silence: shame. He came from a wealthy Jewish background and told one correspondent he was 'born of a couple of rather millionaire lines',[30] and I wonder if part of his reluctance to write about the Depression had something to do with this unspoken inheritance. His father was the son of a diamond merchant, and he was raised in affluent New Rochelle. His little sister grew up to wear furs and pearls,[31] and the family home was a palatial, marble 'non-home' of ornaments and opulence.[32] They had a Japanese butler, a valet and a chauffeur.[33] This monied childhood, of servants and pearls, was at odds with his life as a communist agitator in the 1930s. Even as newlyweds, before the Depression, George and Mary had tried to escape his family's sphere of influence, leaving the country and living under pseudonyms – anything to escape the family name. And so it seems to me that there was always something he was keeping back, an element of his life that remained unsaid. As Mary admitted in a later interview, the couple's financial security was the 'guilty secret' that allowed them to risk arrest on a picket line – as nothing mattered quite as much when you had money.[34]

And there was perhaps something shameful about his financial security in the face of starvation that helped to stop his tongue.

*

It was shame, too, that seeded my silence. I was raised to believe that there are aspects of your life that shouldn't, and couldn't, be talked about. And this shame became almost unbearable the day my father lost his job.

I was told from the start his redundancy was to be kept secret, and overnight he stopped being the bearer of treats and surprises. It must have been around a year after I started secondary school, and to my parents it would have felt as though the world had cracked open. They had a house in the home counties and four sets of school fees to meet – so the loss of his income was unimaginable. In the weeks that followed, it felt as though I was peeping through my fingers at a horror film – unable to see the screen, but knowing something terrible was happening. The house became cold, the empty rooms suddenly dark. My parents' fights became louder, longer. Things were broken. One afternoon I encountered my father crying in the study, pressing his fingers against his eyes, his mouth hanging empty. He turned his chair away as I walked past. We heard doors slam, and my mother would drive off for hours without telling us where she was going.

'Try not to worry,' my father would say. 'It's my fault. She'll be back.'

My father's sudden redundancy changed the shape of home life. In the years that followed, my grandmother arrived to help take care of my younger siblings, and my mother retrained as a teacher – sitting in the living room wrapped in a blanket, reading textbooks, with the curtains closed.

I stopped sleeping. I would lie awake until the early hours worrying about the day ahead, listening to my baby brother screaming. One night I peered into my parents' room looking for comfort.

'What now?' my mother asked. She hadn't yet slept – run ragged by the redundancy, and a toddler, and the prospect of her mother moving in.

My father led me downstairs and we slid on wellies over our cold feet and pyjamas. We walked hand in hand along the lane, beside the house, where he had taught me to ride a bike – running along behind, never telling me when he had let go of the saddle and I was doing it all by myself.

'I'm sorry,' he said, and squeezed my hand. I looked at my wellies. There was nothing to say.

Silence closed over the house, and we were told not to tell anyone outside the family what was going on. In school the other girls went skiing in Verbier and hung out on the King's Road – no one admitted to living off credit cards and crossed fingers.

'Blood runs thicker than water,' my mother had said, as she finished breakfast one morning, 'and people don't need to know about Daddy.'

At school we were learning about the Christian work ethic. The scripture teacher made it sound so simple. 'Consider the lilies of the field,' she told us. 'They neither toil nor spin, yet even Solomon in all his glory was not arrayed as one of these.' It was the first time I had viewed an adult with contempt – her image of unemployment was nothing like the creeping despair in our unheated house. And as she stood at the front of the class, my eyes were level with her crotch, pinched in tight trousers.

'You don't have a fucking clue,' I thought, relishing the weight of the adult expletive. But I said nothing – and so the gulf between home and school grew wider.

My favourite moments were when I didn't have to do anything, and there were no expectations of me. I yearned for the three minutes of silent prayer in chapel every morning when I could sit with my head down in the crook of my arm, the ridges of my jumper embossed on my forehead.

At home I watched as my parents stopped speaking to each other – or answering my questions about what was happening. My father began sleeping in the downstairs bedroom on occasion. I would talk to him, sitting on the floor in the darkness.

'Are you going to get divorced?' I asked.

'I don't know,' he said to the ceiling. I would come back upstairs to my mother and ask the same question. I never got a straight reply.

My siblings don't remember this time of our lives. When I asked my younger brother about the year my father lost his job, his abiding memory was that we had to switch to Value chocolate spread, and that there were no brands any more: the larder was lined with the blue stripe of Tesco basics.

As things deteriorated at home, I couldn't find the words to tell my family what was happening at school: it seemed irrelevant in the face of their sadness. And at school, I knew not to talk about the separate bedrooms and shouting – so I didn't. I took an involuntary step back from the world, and stopped telling anyone how I was feeling.

Once I began to research childhood mutism, I learnt that one of the most powerful indicators of whether a child will stop speaking is the behaviour they see modelled by their parents. The most famous example of childhood mutism en masse involves the children of a remote community in Eastern Kentucky, who stopped speaking when they were forced to switch schools. It began in the winter of 1964, when a squat concrete consolidated high school opened in Big Creek in the Appalachian mountains. The school took in over 300 children who had come from tiny one- and two-classroom village schools in the surrounding hollows and coves. Many of these children had never ventured beyond their rural homesteads, and as the term drew on it became clear that some of them were, to coin the local phrase, 'quiet-turned'. From the moment they boarded the school bus they did not utter a word and would not move to go to the bathroom, lunchroom or playground. Instead they sat silently in their seats.[35]

The psychologist David Looff noted that many of these children were also habitually quiet at home, having observed that their parents valued silence. Many of their fathers earned their living as hunters and ice fishers, and would sit alone on the snow without uttering a word for hours at a time, forming a 'training pattern' that their children would emulate as they sat beside them on the ice. Perhaps in a household that couldn't talk about what was happening, it was inevitable I would slip into silence – or maybe as the daughter of generations of taciturn men, being 'quiet-turned' was simply a hereditary quirk, like colour blindness or sand-blonde hair.

EPILEPTIC THERAPY DOG

IT STARTS TO RAIN AS I leave Leicester station. I hurry up the hill, past the boarded-up houses and chip shops, wishing I had brought an umbrella. I have left too much time, and sidle into a corner shop to stare absently at the headlines. I don't want to be early. I had hoped to slip into the back of the room as the conference started, to avoid the risk of small talk.

This is a dead-end part of town, with its blacked-out windows, empty coffee shops and student digs. There are worn 'Vote Labour' stickers on the letterboxes and cans of cider and Red Bull stacked against the windows, with sheets hung across the glass in place of curtains. Ahead of me I can see other lone female figures, furtively checking their phones to see if they are on course. We don't acknowledge each other.

I am on my way to the annual conference of an organisation dedicated to helping children to find their voices: SMIRA, or the Selective Mutism Information and Research Association. After starting to explore my own silence, I began to read about other children who had lost the ability to speak at will, and came across the term selective mutism in a slightly dated psychology textbook with an image of a small child with their mouth sealed shut with sticking plasters on the cover. As I read, I discovered that when children stop speaking at school it is often due to this misunderstood anxiety disorder, which is thought to affect up to one in every 150 children. It is characterised by the fact that a child with the condition will be unable to speak to certain people in certain situations, most usually in the classroom.[36]

I learnt that initially selective mutism – or SM – can be hard to diagnose, as the child's behaviour may seem quite normal: the toddler clinging to his mother's legs and shying away when asked his name. But while other children adapt to school life and begin to speak – reaching for the Play-Doh and smiling – a selectively mute child may retreat into silence, meeting the world with a blank expression: flat and unreadable, as if they aren't quite there.[37]

I did not stop speaking until I was a teenager, but I recognise myself in the descriptions of selectively mute children – hypersensitive to the demands of the world. When I started nursery, I have been told that I would barricade myself in the Wendy House and refuse to speak to anyone until I went home. And, like many selectively mute children, while I stopped talking at school, I remained articulate and bright at home.

The fact that selectively mute children are often able to speak freely in some settings means that in early studies they were labelled as obstinate, difficult and taciturn. Their silence was mistaken for strong will, rather than fear.[38] I hoped that by coming to the SMIRA conference I would learn more about the condition, and perhaps gain further insight into my own struggles to speak.

Inside, the hall smells of egg mayonnaise and expectation. The event seems to be run mainly by women: one peels cling film from trays of homemade baps; another arranges cups and saucers for the tea break; while a third distributes handwritten name cards.

I take a seat towards the back, beside a woman in a black velour tracksuit, playing Candy Crush on her phone. The silence is punctuated by the tap of acrylic nails on plastic.

'Have you been to one of these before?' she asks.

'No,' I reply.

'Oh, what brings you here, then?' she asks. 'Are you a parent too?'

'No,' I reply, 'I just wanted to find out more about it.' I begin slowly running my finger around the rim of the teacup in my lap, 'Because there was a time when I didn't really talk at school.' I pause – I have never said the words in public before.

'Oh'.

I carry on, trying to preempt the next question, and bring the conversation to a close – leaving no room for questions I can't yet answer.

'I wasn't formally diagnosed with SM,' I continue, barely pausing for breath, 'but I didn't really speak to anyone at school for a while.' I smile. My hand tight on the tea cup.

'Oh,' she says.

A woman at the front of the hall claps her hands to get our

attention – and the woman beside me crosses her legs in the other direction.

'Thank you so much for coming,' the woman at the front begins. 'I think I recognise some of the faces here, but for those of you who don't know me, I'm a speech and language therapist, specialising in the treatment of selective mutism'.

'Now, I'm sure I don't need to tell any of you this,' she continues, with a clipped laugh, 'but selective mutism is a phobia of talking. If someone is suffering from selective mutism – or SM – then they will do anything rather than speak. They might not feel able to ask to use the toilet at school, or tell a teacher if they're hurt.'

The speaker's hair is artificially curled, and she flicks her head to keep the loose waves out of her eyes as she paces to and fro. Layers of chiffon disguise her flesh, leaving no sense of the folds of her body.

'SM can take many forms: sometimes children aren't talking in school – but it could also mean they can't talk to members of their own family.' She stops mid-stride, turning back to face the room, and continues, 'I'm working with one little girl at the moment who hasn't spoken to her dad for five years.' Murmurs of recognition ripple around the room. I take another sip of tea. I didn't know anxiety could become so crippling that it could stop you from crying out in pain, or that silence could seep so deep into the heart of a family. I feel sick. My own experiences seem painfully trivial in the face of this suffering. I want to leave.

*

In the weeks after the conference, I go to visit the speaker at her offices, deep in the Derbyshire countryside. She is called Libby Hill, and is one of only a handful of speech and language therapists in the UK to specialise in treating selectively mute children – who all too often fall into the cracks between mental health services and speech therapists, with no consensus about who should be taking the lead. She is also the owner of the only speech therapy dog in the UK: a chocolate labrador called Ralph. Many of the children she sees find it easier to talk to Ralph than to people – as it is perhaps the safest form of communication. There is no risk that he will answer back, interrupt or say the wrong thing, and working with a speech therapy dog can also help to show children that they have agency in a frightening world. 'It's amazing watching them,' she says, 'and seeing them realise that their voices can make things happen: they can say, "Sit" and "Stay" and "Come here", and he will listen.' For some, working with Ralph is the first time in their lives they will have been heard outside their homes.

But, since being trained, Ralph has developed epilepsy, so the work he can do is now limited, as there is always a chance he will have a fit. Faced with the image of an epileptic therapy dog and a nervous silent child, I stifle an involuntary smile. Despite the advances in treating SM over the years, Libby still sees teenagers who have lived with mutism for so long it has caused irreparable damage. She tells me about one teenager who came to her in desperation, with scarring on her bladder, and kidney damage from repeated urinary tract infections – caused by always holding on when she needed the toilet, as she couldn't ask a teacher if she could be excused.

Back at the SMIRA conference, therapists take notes, and parents raise their hands to describe their children's anxieties and the lengths they would go to in order to avoid speech. One parent explains how her daughter packs and re-packs her school bag late into the night, so she can be sure she won't forget anything and won't need to ask her teacher for help.

I recognise this need to blend in from my own childhood. I would agonise about which posters I should have in my room, so that no one would comment on them, and dreaded being asked my opinion on the bands I listened to – or which member of Take That I was supposed to fancy. Any question without an empirical right answer was dangerous – an opportunity for ridicule.

And yet, as I listen to the parents describing their silent children, I can't be sure if I was ever selectively mute – or simply an anxious child. The key question, one speech therapist tells the room, when trying to decide if a child needs help, is more straightforward: 'Is this child speaking normally? Are they initiating spontaneous social interactions?' At school I never started conversations. I would answer questions – but only when I knew the answer was right – and I clung to the humiliations that punctuated school life: the French class laughing at my pronunciation of 'shampooing', and being made to stand up in a history lesson as my bowl haircut was an illustration of a sixteenth-century 'round head'. The smallest tragedies always outweighed the greatest triumphs.

I leave the conference without speaking to anyone, picking up a leftover egg mayonnaise bap for the train, and walking quickly back down the hill. I could not have imagined that speaking could become so terrifying that you would rather endure permanent scarring on your bladder than risk asking to be excused. There is something compelling about these children who have taken this involuntary step away from the world, from community and connection. I am desperate to talk to them.

HYSTERIA & BLESSED WAX

ONE OF THE MOST INTRIGUING cases of mutism I came across was that of the hysterical mutes, who were treated in nineteenth-century Paris. They were a cause célèbre in the medical world, interred in the Salpêtrière Hospital – so called as it was the old gunpowder, or saltpetre, factory in Paris. They would display strange behaviour, which sat somewhere between psychosomatic and somatic disorders – as their symptoms were both medically inexplicable and physically undeniable. These women captured the public imagination, and are epitomised by a painting in which a woman swoons in a dead faint before an audience of intrigued doctors.[39]

The picture shows a woman named Blanche, who was the self-styled 'queen of the hysterics', and arrived at the Salpêtrière aged eighteen. At the time she was known as Marie Wittman, and her biography is piecemeal, based solely on the accounts of the doctors who recorded her story.[40] According to these notes, her father was a carpenter and her mother a laundress, and Blanche suffered convulsions as a child that left her temporarily deaf and dumb. As a teenager she was sent as apprentice to a furrier, who molested her, until she was eventually hired as a ward girl, working in the laundry of the Salpêtrière to earn her keep.

Once at the hospital, she became the model hysteric, exhibiting symptoms almost on command. Like many patients she suffered a 'globus hystericus' lump in the throat,[41] which would have felt like she was choking, and there were times when she was struck dumb. I am astounded when I read this diagnosis – as I have also suffered from 'globus', as it is now known. It happened a couple of years ago. I had just been made redundant, and after weeks of applying for jobs that did not materialise, I began to feel a tightness in my throat that could only be stilled by sleep. Each morning I would feel it contract as I lay inert waiting for the day to begin. And as the hours passed it coalesced into a physical lump – a hard mass when I tried to swallow. The GP told me there was nothing there: 'It's a common psychological symptom,' she said. 'Are you under undue stress?' She swivelled the computer screen towards me, to show me the name of the complaint 'globus hystericus'. She paused, embarrassed. 'We tend not to say the hystericus bit these days – as it's a bit patronising,' she said. There was, she told me, nothing to be done – it was a psychosomatic symptom. She prescribed some antacid pills and sent me home. But in the nineteenth century doctors engineered increasingly bizarre ways of alleviating these hysterical symptoms and helping patients to recover their voices.

Blanche's bouts of hysterical mutism and paralysis could be brought on, and stopped, using hypnosis or, on occasion, the application of pressure to the ovaries with a machine reminiscent of an instrument of torture. The head doctor at the Salpêtrière, Jean-Martin Charcot, had identified what he called 'hysterogenic zones',[42] including the ovaries and mammary glands, which, according to the historian Asti Hustvedt, were a 'mechanical button of sorts that when pressed could trigger or arrest a hysterical attack'. Charcot's methods were discredited after his death – and Blanche spent the rest of her life in the hospital – eventually working as an assistant to Marie Curie, and losing several limbs as a result of radiation exposure.

But Charcot was not simply an outdated quack; it has been argued that his treatment of hysteria paved the way for psychoanalysis, or the talking cure, which would help so many to break their silence in years to come.[43] Sigmund Freud admired Charcot and had visited the Salpêtrière, and some historians now argue that Freud's initial attempts at psychoanalysis were indebted to Charcot's methods – for both cured their patients through a performance: by encouraging a patient to talk about their experiences, or re-enact them under hypnosis. Rather than performing to an assembled audience of doctors, in Freud's consulting room the talking cure became a 'one-woman show', with the patient both actor and audience.[44]

Charcot is also not alone in his use of strange methodology to treat silence – over the years therapists have resorted to a series of bizarre methods in an effort to get their patients to speak. One of the most unlikely treatments for selective mutism involved the use of a substance known as 'blessed wax', which was used to cure a little boy in Switzerland in 1934. Known only as 'A', he would not speak to teachers during lessons and did not talk to any relatives other than his father. In desperation, 'A's mother sought the help of a 'capuzin monk' during the Easter holidays, who reportedly gave her a block of 'blessed wax' and told her to feed the child small chunks each day. She followed his advice, also sewing the wax into her son's school blazer – and within three weeks 'A' could speak again.[45] The child's recovery was documented by the Swiss doctor Moritz Tramer, who went on to coin the phrase 'elective mutism' to describe the boy's affliction.[46] The term was used by medical professionals for the next sixty years[47] and was eventually cast off in favour of 'selective mutism', to make it clear that children do not choose when and to whom they speak – but are in the grip of paralysing anxiety.

One speech and language therapist, named Maggie Johnson, is particularly renowned for her suggestion that not only is this type of mutism an involuntary response to the expectation to speak, but is in fact best understood as a phobia of talking to certain people. This idea that has revolutionised the way SM is understood and treated in the UK.[48]

I first saw Maggie speak at the SMIRA conference, where she had the air of a celebrity – beautiful, blonde and encircled by admirers. I felt I didn't know enough in those early days to approach her in person, and it took several needling emails before she finally agreed to speak to me. As well as working for the NHS, she is overwhelmed by requests for help from families around the world, and her time is precious.

Like so many of the professionals I have spoken to, Maggie

tells me that her interest in the subject began with failure. She was working in a residential school, and had been sent to see a teenage boy. 'All I was told,' she says, 'was that he wasn't talking, and that I needed to go and make him speak.' As a 'very green' young speech and language therapist she didn't know what to do. 'So I just sat it out – I just sat and stared him out.' The staff at the centre knew that the boy could speak to his mother, so it was assumed that his mutism was something he could pick up or drop at will. Between visits home at the end of term, his only means of communication with his mother was via the public payphone in the corridor, and he was too scared to speak in the open, where he could be overheard. 'So he had devised a code to speak to her – two taps on the receiver meant yes, and one tap meant no – and that was it. That was the only communication he had.'

After weeks of staring at each other, Maggie realised this boy wasn't choosing his silence when she saw a 'huge tear rolling down his face' during a therapy session. 'There was no movement, his face was completely immobile and still,' she says, 'but I was just shocked to the core, and it was only in that moment that I realised: he's not refusing to speak – he's desperate – he knew if he could speak then he could just go home. Everything changed for me in that moment. I still wasn't able to help him. But I knew then that this wasn't deliberate.'

The boy subsequently left the school and when Maggie returned the following term the staff were told he had tried to kill himself. 'It was just devastating,' she says, 'and I vowed I would never let anyone down like that again. From then on it became a personal crusade for me.'

Forty years later, her books are credited with helping countless children recover her voices, and desperate parents will eagerly attend her masterclasses. But the real breakthrough only came about when her six-year-old daughter developed a debilitating phobia of ants – and she realised that selective mutism could also be understood as a phobia of talking. 'It sounds ridiculous,' she says, laughing. 'I mean, how can anybody have a phobia of ants? But when you witness your child hyperventilating and highly distressed over a pathetic ant – you realise you can have a phobia of anything.'

Maggie took her daughter to see a child psychiatrist, who suggested that her daughter's fear stemmed from a holiday in Australia. As Maggie recalls, they were squeezed into the back of a taxi, when a 'disgusting enormous creature' flew through the window and landed on her daughter's back. As they were driving at speed, with no way of escaping the insect, Maggie 'freaked out' and started 'screaming "Stop the car, stop the car!"' After what felt like an impossibly long delay, they were able to pull over, and as they tumbled out of the back seat, Maggie managed to brush the insect off and it flew away. Maggie still doesn't know what the insect was – but when her daughter asked what was wrong, Maggie told her it was 'just a flying ant'. The psychiatrist explained that Maggie's daughter's fear at seeing her mother lose control had been subconsciously attached to the word ant – via a principle known as 'transference'. From that day on, the psychohiatrist said, whenever her daughter saw an ant, the panic of that moment came flooding back to her, so that she had developed a phobia of ants, and now couldn't stand to be near them.

At that moment, Maggie tells me, she had 'this amazing light bulb moment', as she realised this principle of transference could explain why the children she was treating had developed an otherwise inexplicable fear of speaking. And why, despite their desperate desire to talk, they were unable to get the words out. 'Half of me was just crying,' she says, 'and thinking, as a mum, "What have I done to my child?" – and the other half was thinking: "Oh my goodness, this explains everything."'

Phobias originate in what Maggie describes as the 'most primitive' part of the brain, the amygdala, an almond-shaped bundle of nerves, responsible for processing emotions. She explains that when the amygdala processes emotional memories, other parts of the same event – like smells, sounds or objects – can become associated with that emotion. So, for example, if a child is lost and panicking, and someone asks his name, then the act of speaking can be associated with the terror of being lost, and every time they are subsequently asked to speak to someone new the fear comes flooding back.

Once a phobia has developed it is incredibly difficult to overcome, as the amygdala responds to stimulae twenty times faster than the frontal cortex, where logical thought takes place. So, as Maggie explains, 'fear kicks in and the brain goes to panic mode – before reason tells you there is nothing to fear'. The key to treating phobias, Maggie tells me, is teaching the brain that there is no threat, in short to switch off the amygdala. And the best way to do that is through repeated exposure – to face your fear in tiny steps and at your own pace.

'It's a wonderful thing if you overcome a phobia,' she says. 'It's exhilarating – as you're released from this trap you've been in, and you think, "How on earth could I have been scared of that?"'

As she talks, I am reminded of how I tried to break my own silence by telling myself over and over that I needed to speak: 'You are an interesting person,' I would say to myself, standing against the cloaks in the boot room, 'you have things to say. You have things to say.' But, as I listen to her explain transference and phobias, I am uneasy. I didn't have a phobia of speaking per se. I was never scared of reading aloud, for example – it was more that I was endlessly worried about saying the right thing.

The fact that I found some situations easier to speak in than others is very common. When I first saw Maggie speak at the SMIRA conference, she explained that for most children with SM, there is a hierarchy of speaking – with spontaneous conversation provoking the most anxiety, and rote responses the least. And for some children, speaking someone else's words can feel safer than talking, as there is less risk that they will make a mistake and be asked to repeat themselves.

The key, Maggie tells me, is to try and ease the nerves whirring behind the silent face, and approach everything in small steps rather than getting angry and impatient. One method Maggie uses when working with older children is to ask them to call National Rail Enquiries – but only to speak to the automated 'train tracker' initially. This gives them the chance to start to talk if and when they are ready, and to practice overriding their anxiety response. She has also encouraged older children to practise leaving messages on her answering machine – initially when she is out of the house, so there is no risk they will be overhead. This way they can speak at their own pace, and repeat the activity until their anxiety subsides, and the amygdala has learnt that is no threat, and no longer responds in panic mode.[49]

POETRY

MY OWN RECOVERY WAS A slow process – catalysed by my ability to read aloud. At the point things began to change, I hadn't had a normal conversation at school for months and I knew something had to give. I was growing increasingly unhappy and was desperate to find a way to prove I had a voice. I think I hoped that if I could just show everyone I was physically able to speak, then I would somehow jolt myself out of the silence.

I had always been good at reciting poetry as a child – enjoying the pleasing rise and fall of iambic pentameter, long before I knew it had a name – and so I set my sights on the annual speech and drama competition. The idea of reading someone else's words felt far safer than talking.

The finals were held at the end of the summer term, and the whole school gathered in the auditorium to watch. I was due to perform in the evening, at the end of a sticky July afternoon. Everyone had taken off their ties, and the sixth form wore flip-flops with their school skirts.

The leggings and polo neck I was wearing were camouflage

against the black-box stage, leaving me hands and feet and face. I could feel the sweat under my roll neck in a damp runnel down my back, and there was a soft fold of flesh against the waistband of my leggings. I fiddled with an elastic band, wrapping it around my fingers and stuffing it down my sleeve to still the anxiety – a habit I have never quite abandoned.

I knew I could speak someone else's words – and muttered them under my breath, the elastic tacky in my palm. My mother had taken me out of school when I was eight to compete in declamation exams, and had read to me in the slow hours of insomnia when everything else at home was breaking apart. I would fall asleep listening to her speaking in the voices of people that never existed: Moon Face and the Psammead. The words of others were important.

I had chosen the poem from a collection provided by the drama teacher. It was about death – a trauma greater than anything I had experienced – a serious and grown-up loss that mattered. I knew the words by heart.

There was a sign saying 'Finalist' taped to the floor by my seat, and as I stood I could feel my heart in my chest, and the colour spreading across my face. But once I started I was in suspended animation; speaking almost automatically, my voice was clear and strong in the silence of the auditorium.

> Aunt Julia spoke Gaelic
> very loud and very fast.
> By the time I had learned
> a little, she lay

silenced in the absolute black
of a sandy grave
at Luskentyre. But I hear her still, welcoming me
with a seagull's voice
across a hundred yards
of peatscrapes and lazybeds
and getting angry, getting angry
with so many questions
unanswered.[50]

The hall was silent – and the plastic seat still warm when I sat down to watch the older girls perform their pieces. After the competition I stayed the night on a spare bed in one of the dormitories, and counted the glow stars on the ceiling as I listened to other people breathing. It is only looking back that I realise I had gravitated towards a poem about the frustrations of silence – and the anger of coming face to face with the wordless dead.

After the poetry reading I gradually gained in confidence, and began to speak more at school. I still struggled to hold my own in large groups, and found it easier to talk one on one or when there were other activities for distraction, so there was something to return to when the words dried up. It took a long time before friendships felt natural and I could engage in the dance of spontaneous conversation. Many old school friends now say they have no memory of my silence, which of course was the idea – to disappear for a while.

For Oppen, poetry also catalysed the end of his silence, as he was struck by a sudden, urgent, need to write. The story goes that he had a dream, which gave him a sudden and life-changing premonition that he needed to return to his verse. He dreamed that he was going through his father's old filing cabinet and came across notes on how to prevent rust in copper. At the time he thought it was strange, as he presumed that even his father would have known copper could not rust. It was only when he discussed the dream with a therapist that he realised the rust was a metaphor. 'You are worried that you yourself are going to rust,' the therapist reportedly told him. The thought of his poetic talent going to waste was, apparently, enough to spur him on to buy pencils and paper on the way home from the therapist's office, and to begin writing the very same day.[51]

This story is repeated in Mary's autobiography, and in interviews given in the years after Oppen's silence. And as I read the accounts of this Damascene moment, I am disappointed. It seems too simple. How could over two decades of silence come down to a dream? Surely it would take more to find his voice – especially given that by the time Oppen had this dream, his commitment to silence had driven him far from home – to the life of a political exile.

Oppen's connections to the Communist Party, forged in the despair of the Depression, eventually resulted in him having to leave America, as he fell under the suspicion of Senator McCarthy and the House Un-American Activities Committee (HUAC). Although George and Mary's main period of involvement in the Communist Party was over by 1941,[52] the Oppens did not hand in their Party membership cards, which, coupled with their support of the Wallace presidential campaign, was enough to raise the alarm and send the FBI to their door. At the time McCarthy was intent on eliminating the red threat, and anyone suspected of communist sympathies was liable to be interrogated or imprisoned. The FBI visited the Oppens' house in California several times in the late 1940s, and Linda, George's daughter, remembers being told never to speak to men who called at the house with white folded handkerchiefs in their breast pockets.[53] By this point, as Mary explained in a letter, it was not easy to leave the Party, and so, rather than risk imprisonment and leave a young child without her parents, or to have to name names – the family fled to Mexico, where they lived from 1950 to 1958.[54]

Mary recounts in her autobiography how they drove through searing heat to the border, trying to revive Linda's pet parakeet, who was wilting in the desert sun.[55] They entered Mexico hoping to live with local people, and not be confined to a group of émigrés – but life didn't turn out that way. The family were laid low with food poisoning as soon as they arrived, with George fainting in the hotel bathtub after the long desert drive. According to Mary's account, they were sick several times during these early months, and a horror of drinking the water or eating homemade food made it difficult to mix with local people.[56] In their first few years in Mexico, the Oppens also realised they were being watched, and on more than one occasion were interrogated by two men who seemed to have access to the information held on the Oppens by the FBI.[57] Although these interrogations stopped when a local lawyer got involved, they were enough to persuade George and Mary of the need to watch what they said – and they adapted their lives accordingly.

The family had chosen Mexico as it was one of the few places they could access by road without a passport. But, once there, they could not safely return home until they were granted US passports, and thus did not feel their lives were their own. Linda Oppen remembers this as a time of sadness in her parents' lives[58] – and it was also marked by secrecy, as the couple made a conscious decision not to talk about their past life, having learnt from experience that you never knew who was watching and listening. Alongside this, they also actively concealed George's work as a poet and instead built a life as artisans: George learnt carpentry and managed a furniture business, while Mary painted. But the secrets caused rifts between them and their fellow émigrés – Mary recalls in her autobiography that one friend made during the Mexico years was deeply affronted when she found out that George had been a poet – and was known to William Carlos Williams.[59]

Into this came George's dream about rust in copper. But it was not simply the dream that changed things – international events also conspired to make it easier for Oppen to begin writing again. The Oppens' application for American passports was finally approved in 1958, seven years after they had first applied, and they were at last able to go back to the US, so that Linda could enrol at college. Back in California, with Linda away studying, the Oppens were no longer full-time parents – or political exiles – and had agency over their lives once more. It was these changes, as well as the catalytic dream, which allowed Oppen to return to his work.

Almost as soon as Oppen arrived back in the US he began sending poems to friends and publishers, in the hope of taking up where he had left off decades earlier. In those frenzied first years he would write for up to eight hours a day, seemingly to make up for lost time – and what is apparent, in his daybooks, his letters, his poetry, is how seriously he took the act of writing after his years of silence. Oppen's day books, the working documents from which he constructed his poetry, show how these new poems were built from the rubble, through endless revision. The pages of the books were physically held together with whatever came to hand, sometimes pipe-cleaners, and in one case were nailed to a block of wood. The poems grew out of autobiographical notes, shopping lists, drafts of letters – all given space on the page.[60]

What is interesting is that for a poet who turned his back on writing for so long, Oppen gives great weight to the 'little words', once he started writing again. The words he chooses are important, weighed and measured against each other, to the extent that he called one collection of poetry *This is Which* – the title calling our attention to the connective tissue, the conjunctions and prepositions which are normally glossed over. In an interview in the 1960s, Oppen said that these 'little words I like so much' are 'crying faith' in the fact that the world exists, and that language is able to refer to, and communicate, that physical reality. Poetry is, in short, 'a test of truth'.[61] 'You say these perfect little words,' he says, 'and you're asserting that the sun is ninety-three million miles away . . . and there is more, who knows? It's a tremendous structure to have built out of a few nouns.'[62]

Once he began writing again, his poems become imbued with this deep sense of wonder at both the physical reality of the world and the mechanism of language, in allowing us to describe and express our experience. I recognise this relief – that language works. It is the delight of the child watching the therapy dog canter towards them, as they asked him to 'come', or the pleasure of sharing a confidence with a friend – the sheer delight that the world exists, and that through language we are able to participate in it.

GROWING UP

In HINDSIGHT I WAS LUCKY that the acute period of my speechlessness passed within a year. Many cannot say the same, and although SM usually responds well to treatment, if the condition is left untreated then the emptiness of a silent childhood can pave the way to a troubled adult life.[63]

Many of the selectively mute adults I have spoken to have developed other mental health issues, like OCD, social phobias and depression.

I spend weeks contacting support groups and forums, hoping to glimpse the daily life of the selectively mute – but they are elusive. Many people offer to help, but the vast majority will only communicate via email, as the phone provokes too much anxiety. They are slight, shadowy figures – connected by Facebook groups and yet chronically isolated. They send voluminous emails, and yet, sending me their stories fully formed, without the mediation of spoken questions, feels like a way of shutting down the conversation and asserting some form of control. It is a frustrating process, and I glimpse the exasperated teacher berating the silent child in my reactions. Silence distorts relationships, and I am used to being in control – telling and rebuilding other people's stories as a journalist. They won't let me.

And yet, many speak of feeling powerless, like children. One sufferer, Oliver*, who is now in his twenties, tells me he had friends on the football field at school who never asked for social interaction, but now he is confined to his bedroom and unable to leave the house without his mother to speak for him. 'I feel so much younger than I am,' he tells me via email. 'I'm at an age where everything should be changing, but I am still so dependent on other people.' As he has got older, Oliver has found it harder to communicate, and his selective mutism now means that at times he is unable to communicate non-verbally either. 'When I'm nervous or put on the spot, I'll freeze,' he says. This often happens during therapy, and 'It's incredibly frustrating, and I feel even more trapped within myself – completely useless.' Worryingly, many of the adult SM sufferers I speak to echo his concern that their silent paralysis is getting worse. Jenni is also in her twenties, and now suffers from progressive mutism. She dips in and out of communication, and at the point she emails me, is unable to speak to anyone, including her immediate family. The only way she has found to communicate is using the written word, or by speaking 'through her rabbit', Betsy.

---

* All names of children and young people with SM have been changed to protect their identities.

Eventually I arrange to meet a mother who is willing to talk in person about her almost grown-up children. They are twins, and at the time we meet, are not able to speak to anyone apart from each other. Twins are more likely than other siblings to suffer from selective mutism, and I am nervous about meeting her, having read many disturbing accounts of mute twins during my research. One of the most notorious cases of selective mutism, historically, was that of the 'Silent Twins', June and Jennifer Gibbons, who were committed to Broadmoor as teenagers in the 1980s for arson – and spoke only to each other in a strange patois that even their parents could not understand. As young children the Gibbons twins did not speak at school, and as they grew they withdrew from their family, speaking only occasionally to their younger sister. At primary school one teacher described them as 'like bits of straw in the eddies of a stream . . . always apart from everyone else trying to be invisible'.[64]

As part of the only black family in a small town in Wales, the twins were already socially isolated, and would communicate by leaving notes around the house asking their mother for things they needed. According to their biographer, Marjorie Wallace, their silence was only broken by the death of the older twin, Jennifer, in 1993 following a sudden and inexplicable inflammation of the heart while being transferred from Broadmoor. The surviving twin, June, now lives in Wales and speaks completely normally.

While the Gibbons twins captured the public imagination, it now seems unlikely that they suffered from true selective mutism, as they were not phobic of speech. Rather, their silence was, according to their biographer, an elaborate 'childhood pact', or a sinister 'game', which could be picked up at will[65] – and I was curious to see how modern-day mute twins fared in comparison.

I meet Susannah in an ice-cream parlour one Friday evening. It is warm inside and the backs of my legs are sticky against the polished red banquette. Whenever I stop and make eye contact she freezes, and stirs her melting milkshake, lifting and dropping the blueberries at the bottom of the glass with a plastic spoon.

Her twin daughters, Ann and Lucy,[66] have just celebrated their birthday, and she tells me they all drove to a department store in a taxi for the twins to look at the toys, before coming home for fruit, speared with birthday candles. The twins' anxiety is so severe that they would not let anyone see them open their mouths. They turned away to eat their strawberries, and their younger cousin had to blow the candles out.

Ann and Lucy have now been moved out of mainstream education and are attending a residential school, but come home at the weekends. When they are home, Susannah tells me, they will only speak to each other using a form of sign language that they have invented, and that only the twins understand. If they want to talk to their mother, they will tap out a message on their iPad. It's a frustrating process: 'When they're not in a good mood, they won't communicate at all,' Susannah tells me. 'If I go into their bedroom, they will cover themselves with a blanket, so it's all on their terms. If I come to them and ask something, they get annoyed.'

As is the case with many adult mutes, the twins' predominant emotion is anger. 'When they are frustrated, they can't explain what's gone wrong,' Susannah goes on, taking a sip of her milk-shake. 'I never know if they are in pain – or if they've had a fight among themselves. Then they start trying to sign to me, and I don't understand and get it wrong, and they get very frustrated. What I miss is that we can never deal with these issues by talking. These moments are never resolved. They stay somewhere buried inside.'

The family came to the UK as refugees, and Susannah says the twins grew up knowing that words had to be rationed. 'We never wanted to be heard speaking a foreign language on the street,' she says, 'we were always worried about people listening' – just as George Oppen was always on the lookout for the FBI in Mexico. The twins were also – like many bilingual children – slow to speak, and by the age of four could only say one or two words at a time. Worried, Susannah contacted her GP and set in train a lifetime of referrals to psychologists, psychiatrists, speech and language therapists, and local authority funding tribunals. The younger twin was found to be on the autistic spectrum, and both girls were diagnosed as selectively mute – but after years of careful therapy at primary school were able to talk normally.

However, things began to deteriorate when the girls started secondary school. As their peers began talking about boys, and experimenting with make-up, the twins stopped speaking. Susannah tells me how they were given lockers at the start of term to store their books, but they didn't know the combination to open them. Rather than asking, the twins would carry all their books across town, to and from school each day, until they were physically stooped with anxiety. And rather than ask to use the toilet they would wet themselves on the way home, running along the high street until it was too late. But the school insisted there was nothing wrong, as they were able to pass their exams. Susannah is still furious at the missed opportunities to help: 'There are no words, but there is a voice which must be heard,' she says. 'Those girls, they scream for help without saying a single word. When they walk down the street with their heads down, and people look at them, what is that, if not a cry for help?'

Susannah believes their silence is a way of stopping the forward-spin of the world, and trying to avoid growing up. The younger twin, Ann, says she is 'mute for life'. 'She doesn't want to change,' Susannah tells me, 'and until she does, there is nothing that can be done.' For now, they are totally dependent on their mother when they are at home, and the trio are increasingly cut off from the world. 'I can't leave them,' Susannah tells me. 'What if there was a fire? Would they say anything?'

She shows me pictures of the girls on her phone. They are slight, sylph-like figures, messing around in onesies and baseball caps. The pictures are always taken into a mirror rather than straight-on. Susannah tells me the twins won't let her take photos of them now, as they retreat further and further from the world.

As I travel home, I think of Susannah going back to her empty flat and getting ready for the twins' next visit – tidying their room and making the beds. I have a sense now of what silence does to a family; how it drives people apart and distorts intimacy. But I am growing increasingly aware that I have not yet spoken to anyone first-hand who suffers from selective mutism. Perhaps I am aiming for the impossible, in trying to speak to the silent. But the more I learn about the condition, the more I want to talk to survivors.

And, eventually, I finally have the chance.

SPEAKING OF SOGGY FRIES

I AM IN NEW YORK. The air is so heavy with humidity I can almost hold it. It is 7.45 a.m. and I have a breakfast interview booked across town. I drag the camera kit, lenses, lights and tripod into the waiting Uber. I am exhausted before I have even begun. I have managed to get permission to film a documentary at the first week-long intensive therapy camp for teenagers with selective mutism, and I am excited to finally spend time with selectively mute children. The camp is called WeSpeak, and was set up in 2016, as the organisers were overwhelmed with requests for help for older children. There were already similar camps for pre-schoolers – the crassly titled Mighty Mouth Kids and Brave Buddies – but nothing for children on the cusp of adolescence who, rather than gaining in confidence and independence, were, like Susannah's twins, turning further and further from the world.

There is nothing like WeSpeak in the UK – perhaps because there's something specifically American about sending your children away for the summer. Before I set out for New York I come across a video on YouTube, taken at the sister camp for much younger children. In the video a little girl has to order some food from a play shop, and is so anxious that she wets herself. This seems to be the antithesis of treating SM in the UK, where the key is to minimise the child's anxiety by encouraging them to face their fear in smaller steps, so that each success shows the brain that the fear is not rational, and their physical symptoms subside.

In New York, it seems to me that the kids are pushed to speak. The camp's slogan is 'Get Comfortable With Being Uncomfortable!' and as the founder of the psychology practice that facilitates the camp Dr Steven Kurtz explains, far from eliminating anxiety from the kids' lives, he believes children need to learn to live with fear. 'Our goal is not to treat the anxiety,' he tells me. 'If you talk to adults who have lived with any anxiety disorder, long term, they will tell you that they're constantly having to do exposures. It's a lifestyle.'

The 'exposure lifestyle' is essentially exposing yourself continually to the things that make you uncomfortable. The thinking at WeSpeak is that selective mutism is both the product of a genetic disposition towards anxiety, and also years of learnt behaviour, where a child has become adept at avoiding the situations that make them fearful. Often, Dr Kurtz tells me, their parents will have become unwitting enablers – helping the child to remain mute. He gives the example of a mother who habitually answers for her child whenever a stranger asks them a question. Although she may think she is helping, she is in fact teaching the child that there is no need to talk, as the parents will always come to the rescue. Changing this behaviour is,

Dr Kurtz suggests, inevitably unpleasant and frightening. But the feeling of discomfort is, if anything, an indication that you're doing it right. It can look painful – wrong, even – pushing a child until they are so scared they wet themselves, but feeling afraid can be a strange cipher of success.

This 'exposure' method has been developed over years of working with silent children. One of Dr Kurtz's earliest patients – and success stories – is a boy called Jon, who is now one of the mentors at the WeSpeak camp.[67] His hair is cut into a monastic-looking bowl and he wears the same clothes every day: a uniform of black jeans and T-shirt. Ironically, by trying to blend in, he stands out from the other mentors in their shorts and sneakers. He arrives earlier than anyone else, walking around the corner of the block with a soda at 7.30 a.m., and is observant in the ways I have seen other selectively mute kids to be, as they need to navigate the world without asking for help. He often meets me outside the camp in the mornings, and will offer to carry my camera. He sees me sweating with the weight while others walk past. He notices where would be a good spot for an interview, and has mapped the quiet corners of the building. I am grateful for his attention. It is strange filming on my own: I feel peripheral to the world. The parents are all intent on their children's progress, and no one really asks anything about me. I am staying in the cheapest room of a cheap hotel downtown. The window looks out onto a wall, and it is perennially dark. I end each day sitting under the air conditioning unit in my room, watching the footage and trying to make sense of the children's lives.

Jon explains the challenges for kids with SM well: 'Everyone is like a rat or a spider for these kids,' he says. 'If you're arachnophobic you'll look at a picture of a spider, and you'll still be scared. Even though it's just a picture. It's like that for these kids. They probably can't explain why they feel the way they do, but for them every person is like that spider.' The world he describes is a terrifying place. It reminds me of living in a mansion block in South London, which was overrun by foxes. The only way to get rid of them was to raise your fist as if you were about to throw a rock. It didn't matter if the rock was there or not – the fear was always real – and they would scamper away into the darkness.

On the first day of the camp, the children are physically shielded from the rats and spiders of the world. Each is paired with a mentor who sits beside them, to encourage them to talk. They are in their mid-twenties, and hunched in child-sized chairs. They arrive drinking frappés, and Diet Coke, and are assigned a new kid each morning, so that the children get used to speaking to as many new people as possible. The mentors are impossibly upbeat, excited by the smallest, almost imperceptible triumphs. If a child is able to answer a question, they are immediately praised: 'Well done; good job; great loud voice; thanks for telling me that!' They all turn towards their small charges, so it is physically hard to see the children's faces from my perch at the side of the room. They have an almost meditative awareness of their mentees – following each flinch and murmur – and by the end of the day they are grey-faced and exhausted. Their encouraging chatter is non-stop – and hits you like a surge of water when you enter the room.

I was not expecting the noise. There are no pauses in conversation. No ebb and flow – just sound. The mentors talk in a seemingly continuous stream, congratulating and commenting on everything that is said. It is overwhelming – and I step outside. The hallway is dark and the air almost gelatinous. In the next-door room I can hear small children singing. It is a parallel camp teaching maths and science to pre-schoolers. They run out occasionally to go the bathroom, in matching purple T-shirts. I am always staggered when they say 'Hey!' It is such a simple gesture, and yet so far from the lives of the WeSpeak kids.

These are children who are adept at communicating without speaking. One girl sits silently, with frizzy blonde hair pulled into plaits. She presses her lips together, wide-eyed, begging the mentor to understand. This is Lucinda. She has travelled from Canada with her parents to attend the camp. She is here because she will only speak in a whisper at school. Her parents tell me they first realised something was wrong during a family holiday in Thailand. There, Lucinda fell into a stream and, rather than crying out, she lay inert as a stone, while the water lapped over her face. 'That's when you really worry,' her mother confesses, 'because she couldn't cry out for help. She can't keep herself safe.' She remembers another occasion a few years later, when Lucinda missed the school bus home. Rather than ask a teacher for help, or to use the school phone to call her parents, she decided the best course of action was to walk home. She was found by a neighbour, wandering along the freeway. As I talk to her parents in the cafeteria one afternoon, shouts from the playground drift through the open window. Her dad laughs. 'That's all we want,' he says, 'to hear her playing.' They tell me they can't think of the long term – college and boyfriends and jobs. For now, all they want is for her to make some friends.

What's baffling is that Lucinda talks normally at home. Before the week began, each child had to submit a video introduction, which was played to the class, as the children couldn't introduce themselves in person. The child in Lucinda's video is almost unrecognisable. In the video she sits on the edge of a sofa and talks freely to the camera. She names the animals on the farm – a horse called Adam and the chickens 'which we don't bother naming, as there's no point' – and lists her favourite TV shows, laughing as she recalls a Monty Python skit. But in the classroom she will never raise her voice above a whisper.

The pinnacle of Lucinda's week is reading aloud to the class. She is in a group of girls, each reading a paragraph from an old *National Geographic*.

'Louder,' her mentor says, pushing her chair back from the table so she is a few feet away, 'I can't hear you.'

'The potato chip was invented by accident by George Crum,' Lucinda begins, hands pressed flat against the magazine, 'after a customer complained about soggy fries.'

'Let's do the the last word again.'

'Soggy fries –'

'Again . . .'

'Soggy fries.' She is almost crying – pushing down onto the table so hard her fingers are white. She has not broken out of a whisper.

'Great job!' Her mentor sits back down beside her and Lucinda visibly crumples, folding back in on herself. It is over. Her mentor tells me later that this was the first time Lucinda had ever read aloud in a school setting – and yet I wonder how much use this declaration will be? How will whispering about soggy fries enable her to make friends? It is, I am told by one of the psychologists running the week, simply a small step, and the hope is that each of these steps will help her to build her confidence and eventually regain her voice. As the camp's founder Dr Shelley Avny explains, 'The treatment for anxious kids is to put them in situations that make them anxious, and actually facing their fears. We need them to experience the anxiety in these situations and get through it for them to see that they can.' She continues, 'we'd love to get Lucinda out of her whisper, but her whisper is really secondary. The first step is just getting them talking.'

Other children are already able to speak when the course begins, and I find myself drawn to a little girl who never takes off her backpack. She sits with it hooked over the back of her chair, with the straps tight around her shoulders. She is called Zoe, and is the oldest child in the group and, unlike Lucinda, is able to answer direct questions. 'I like having my stuff,' she tells me, when I ask about the backpack, 'I don't want other people to have it.' I can't question the logic. In many ways she reminds me of myself. At school I would often carry an enormous bag of books through the corridors, in case I needed anything. I rarely read them. There was just something comforting about having them with me.

At first she seems to be streets ahead of the other children, as she is able to answer her mentor's questions, but as I listen,

I notice she will only ever give monosyllabic answers, offering just a few words at a time. She never pauses to consider her responses – as soon as her mentor asks a question she replies. It is almost as though silence is the spider to be chased from the room. She leaves no room for consideration. She never elaborates. She is precise.

'Do you like frozen yoghurt?'

'No.'

'Have you seen the Statue of Liberty?'

'Yes.'

There are no shades of grey, and she never proffers an opinion. When asked which is her favourite *Harry Potter* movie, she shrugs, 'I don't know'. She is ironically most verbose when I ask about her selective mutism.

'Zoe,' I begin, 'could you tell me what it's like when you want to talk but you can't?'

She pauses, uncharacteristically, and wrinkles her nose. 'It's like the words get stuck in my throat,' she says. 'I want to say them, but sometimes I just can't.' Zoe has been on medication for years, and is well versed in the language of therapy. She knows she has 'anxiety' – and at one point in the week says she wants 'tools' to control it. Her mother tells me that Zoe does what she needs to get by at school: she can do class presentations and answer the teachers' questions, but she has struggled to build relationships. Her aim for the week is to learn the dance of conversation, so that she can begin to make friends.

As the week goes on, the children move from fixed-choice questions to developing more elaborate conversations. 'So,' the psychologist leading the group begins one morning, 'if I were to say, "I'm going on holiday next week!" what could you say back?' The children murmur to their mentors, before one raises her hand: 'Where are you going?' 'Great job!' the psychologist replies – and so it continues – with the children offering possible answers, until they have stitched together a conversation. As I watch, part of me wishes I had had this – the impossibly complex art of building relationships broken down into its component parts – while part of me thinks it's absurd to assume you can reduce human interaction to a mathematical formula: question, question, statement. How do you teach the pauses in conversation? Ironically no one explains to the children how to use silence.

The highlight of Zoe's week is a 'conversation' between her and two other girls. They are alone in one of the classrooms. The mentors wait eagerly outside. They practise the skills they have just learnt: question, question, statement.

Zoe sits with her backpack in her lap, a makeshift barricade.

'Do you like to be indoors or outdoors?' she asks, after an impossibly long pause.

'Inside,' one girl replies.

'Why do you like to be inside?' Zoe continues, reaching out into the empty room. My heart goes out to her. No one will help her; the slow factual extraction, which passes for conversation, is driven entirely by her.

'I like to sit inside and watch TV,' the girl replies.

After a pause, Zoe says to the room, 'I like to be outside.' But no one acknowledges her statement.

There is something so sad about all this. I know the girls are desperate to make friends, and yet they don't seem able to elicit basic information from each other, much less build interest or empathy into their words. The conversation hobbles on. Without daily practice, they grasp at topics like leaves in a stream, exchanging information, but never quite conversing. They learn how many floors there are in each other's houses, and how each of them likes to travel: by car or by plane.

I know there are no causes for this. I know and yet I wonder. How did they become scared of the sound of their own voices? I am drawn to one of the only boys in the class, Alex. He is the most severe case they have ever seen at WeSpeak. His mum tells me he is a typical boy at home, who likes playing video games and horse riding. But here he is swamped by anxiety. I can hardly see him. He is physically hidden behind his hand, which springs up to cover his mouth every time he goes to speak.

'I feel like this is our last chance,' his mother tells me. She has a beguiling Southern lilt and fiddles with a gold chain around her neck as she speaks, lifting it and dropping it into her lap. 'No one knows about SM where we're from,' she continues, 'so there is no one who can help.' She lives in the Southern states with her two boys and her husband. She has seen many psychologists. But talking therapy doesn't work with a silent child. She is exasperated: 'They don't know what to do with him, so it's sort of just thirty minutes of wasted time, while somebody tries to talk to them and they're getting no feedback.'

Alex will only communicate with his parents, maternal grandparents and his brother. With teachers he is almost mute. 'He will communicate if you ask him a question,' his mother tells me, 'like, "Do you want the story about the whale, or do you want the story about the sharks? One for whales, two for sharks", and he will hold up fingers for one or two, but that's the extent of communication at school.'

His silence is like a black hole that sucks everything towards itself. His parents' lives have changed to accommodate his SM. His mother now partially home schools him, tutoring him at home and sending him to class to have the assignments marked. The sphere of her life is small: mornings at home with Alex and a walk with her parents and him in the afternoon. She says she doesn't want to see people because they will ask about Alex. And he is angry. After days when he says almost nothing in class he will come home morose and vengeful. 'Seeing him struggling is hard,' she says, 'because you're watching this child who I know can talk, and he just can't get it out. I've asked him before, you know, "Where are your words? Why can't you get your words out?" And he'll say, "They're stuck in my head, I can't get it out."' She continues, 'We just feel like we're at a point where he's going into middle school and every year he seems to be more withdrawn and speaks less.'

His mother tells me how when Alex was two, at pre-school, he shut down and couldn't walk around the classroom. He had once been sick to his stomach at school and threw up across his workbooks. He sat there looking at the cold vomit, without saying a word. One of the other children had had to call the teacher over. Like Lucinda, he couldn't ask for help. And it is this isolation that tears his mother apart: 'I wish he could have a friend,' she tells me. 'I mean, can you imagine going through life without a friend?'

I don't tell her that I do know, all too well, what it feels like to move through the day without friends. When I began to break my silence at school, it wasn't because I wanted to talk particularly – it was just that I couldn't face being alone all the time. I needed companionship. I remember that in the weeks after the poetry-speaking competition, as I gained in confidence, I became more calculating about who I would speak to – picking off the socially powerful girls, as I knew that if I befriended them, then their retinue of admirers would follow. Looking back, it was this need for human contact that outweighed my social anxiety and the fear of talking, or looking stupid, and getting it wrong. After the last day's filming, I watch back the images of Alex as I sit under the whir of the air conditioning, eating handfuls of M&Ms. Perhaps, I think, it is the same for the WeSpeak kids – that it isn't any particular therapeutic intervention that will force them to talk, they simply need to reach a point when it's worth struggling into the silence, with inane questions about being indoors or outdoors, because at least that's the beginning of a human connection.

I had come to WeSpeak expecting to disapprove of the 'exposure' method, of forcing children to face their fears. I thought it seemed cruel and completely contrary to the methods practised by speech therapists in the UK, who advocate trying to remove the pressure to talk, and allow the children to move in small steps at their own pace, and in so doing decrease, rather than increase, the child's anxiety. But for some of these children at least, it seemed to work and all of the parents I spoke to told me that they were delighted with their children's progress after a week at the camp. And there was something deeply moving about watching them take their first tentative steps out into the world. The first conversation between Zoe and the other girls was unbearably stilted, but it was a start, however small – a turning towards the world in trepidation, and saying Yes. Perhaps if they had waited for the anxiety to subside they would have never spoken – and the only way for them to break to silence was to just start: to jump into the world, terrified, and talk, in spite of their fear.

On my last night in New York, I treat myself to dinner in an Italian restaurant around the corner from my hotel, in central Manhattan. The long hours of filming have left me feeling detached from the world. I have not had a conversation with anyone about anything, apart from the film, for a week, and I want to be back in the hum of civilisation. As soon as I order, a British couple at the next table lean across to make conversation. They comment on my accent, and ask what has brought me to the city, and if I am travelling alone. When I explain about WeSpeak, and filming the children who are scared of speaking, they are intrigued.

'How strange,' the woman says. She is wearing white eyeshadow, which is caked into the creases around her eyes, and her wrists are heavy with white and gold bangles. 'I mean,' she continues, 'you've got to blame the parents, don't you?' She leans across, to lay a hand on my table, conspiratorially. 'I mean, something must have gone terribly wrong for a child to stop talking?' I am speechless. The parents I have seen would do anything to help their children, driving for miles from rural Canada and working at two jobs to pay for the therapy. 'I'm not sure it's as simple as that,' I say and ask for the check.

As I wait for my change I think back to the first session of the week. The terrified eyes of the children, and Zoe fiddling with a strand of hair, wrapping and unwrapping it around her fingers. It is such a human need to be able to communicate. I imagine the WeSpeak kids packing up their homework from the week and driving home. Staring out of the window as the world changes around them. I wonder how they will cope away from the camp – how they will survive the new school semester. Will this be the term that they finally speak to other students in their class? I couldn't say. I worry for them; a place at WeSpeak costs several thousand dollars, although some places are offered at subsidised rates and almost every parent I spoke to referred to it as a 'last chance'. What happens if it doesn't work – would it be possible for them to claw their way back into the world, after years of silence?

I collect my change and leave. Outside tourists wearing sandals walk hand in hand, stopping to film the yellow cabs racing past. Businesswomen grab late-night sushi on the way home. The city moves onwards. Spending time at WeSpeak has confirmed to me that I did not have SM as a child – I think I was simply quietened by the shame of my father's redundancy, and unable to find my feet at secondary school. But in a sense, the name given to the condition feels irrelevant. For what the week has given me is a new-found respect for silence – and an understanding that it can seep insidiously into adult life, never to be broken.

PART TWO

SEX

HYDE PARK

IT IS ALMOST IMPOSSIBLE TO end a relationship in a rowing boat. On the most obvious level, there is nowhere to go. We faced each other, helpless, the boat spinning slowly.

'What?' my girlfriend said as she leant back to pull the oars towards her. It was not yet summer and her hands were pink with cold. Water ran along her wrists, and down to the floor of the boat. My feet were wet. I was wearing the wrong shoes.

There was something absurd about all of this – the foam life-vests meant it was impossible to turn or lean in towards each other. So we sat, propped like bookends, with nothing between us. She insisted we should wear them. When we hired the little boat she had laughed, pulling the vest over her shoulder, 'Safety first, especially at sea!'

Of course we weren't at sea. But I was grateful for the humour. My throat was tight, and I could feel the muscles in my face as we waited by the water.

We hired the boats in late spring, nearly two years before my grandmother died. There were other couples on the water, and we looked on as they struggled out of the wooden pier by the Serpentine – splashing and laughing. A wide-eyed child with a Mr Whippy watched us as her father reversed a pedalo out into open water – white fluid running over her fingers. The water churning beneath them.

It was the first weekend we had spent together for weeks. For the past three months I had dipped in and out of our lives, while I filmed overseas on a TV series about women's rights. And although I was now home, I hadn't quite settled back into our life together. I remained strangely absent – physically distant during those days of closed-mouth kisses. But neither of us said anything. I think we hoped if we ignored the problem long enough it would simply go away.

The sun was warm on my back as we pulled away from the pier. I held my bag on my lap to keep it dry while she took the oars, pulling against the weight of water, until the sounds from the shore softened.

There was something reassuring about the slap of wood on water, and the lull of forward motion. It felt safer here than at home. Perhaps because there was nowhere to go, nothing to do but listen.

'I think we need to talk,' I said quietly. The sun flared on the water, and she was thrown off-kilter. The oars knocked against the boat.

'What?'

I swallowed, steadying myself with one hand as the boat swayed. 'I'm not sure this is working.'

The boat spun slowly as she let the oars rest. As we turned,

I squinted against the sun. I knew I needed to say something – and I talked quickly, watching an empty ice-cream wrapper floating near us. 'Ever since I got back from the last filming trip,' I said, 'I haven't felt comfortable at home. I'm just not sure this is the right thing to be doing.'

'What do you mean, the right thing to be doing?'

'I've just been feeling really unsure,' I continued, 'unsure about everything.' I didn't look directly at her as I spoke. I was pleased to be holding my bag in front of me. Glad of its solid weight. A dark tide line rose up my skirt, as it leached the water from around my feet.

She asked me questions I couldn't answer, and I scraped at the paint on the side of the boat with my thumbnail. I wished we were on the shore, so I could walk away. Or lie beside her, quietly, and feel the length of her against me.

But nothing fitted together cleanly, and she was clumsy as she tried to balance the oars against the side to pull her sunglasses off and wipe her eyes. I wanted to help.

'I'm so fucking angry,' she said, as she wiped her sunglasses against her shirt. 'I feel so stupid . . .'

'Please don't feel stupid. It's –'

'Do you love me?' She was looking at me now. Her face in shadow as the boat turned. The muscles in her neck were taut as she tried to hold her mouth steady. She looked so sad.

'Yes.'

'Do you love me as much as I love you?'

I didn't answer. She started rowing again, pulling furiously against the water, which splashed cold into the boat.

*

The argument comes back to me as I walk back through Hyde Park after an editorial meeting. A group of Spanish teenagers are reading the Lonely Planet entry on the Serpentine aloud to each other as they walk along the cycle path, and men in Lycra race past on their bikes. It is early evening and the air is cold. The little boats are chained up by the pier, and the blocks and spikes of the London skyline are picked out against the reddening sky.

Ever since meeting the kids at WeSpeak, I have been thinking about the effect that silence has on you in the long term. How does it distort the features of your life? From speaking to those who were silent in childhood, I know it can leave a strange and lasting legacy. One woman I spoke to, who had selective mutism until she was in her forties, told me that she was still excellent at map-reading, as she was so accustomed to finding her way around without asking directions. Even now, after years of speaking normally, she will still try and find her own way rather than asking for help.

Now I have started to look for it, I can see the effects of my early silence throughout my life. I am most aware of it in relationships – the spaces where you should be doing the most intimate communication. I have often found that speech has let me down, and I am left adrift – spinning slowly with nowhere to go.

Perhaps it is a legacy from my schooldays. I started boarding after three years as a day girl, as I hoped it would be a better way to make friends. And it was – most of my school life was very happy. I was head of house. I got straight As. I did well. But I became adept at being with people and yet always at one remove. I never switched off or relaxed entirely and was always slightly on guard. At school I never found the absolute safety of a childhood bedroom. Sometimes I think that being at boarding school was a prototypical version of social media: we were never alone, always observed, judged, validated by the gaze of others. And that does something strange to your sense of self.

As I grew, and started to form romantic relationships, the holding back continued. I subconsciously kept something of myself safe, and silent. I found it hard to articulate what I was feeling. I would worry things were going to go wrong, but would be unable to express this – somehow unsure how to start a conversation that could upset the status quo. And that is how I found myself on a rowing boat in Hyde Park, breaking apart a relationship that had lasted two years.

My girlfriend and I had been living together for six months at the point we hired the boat. The move had come at a time of profound upheaval. I had been made redundant just before we moved in together, and I was still finding my way around the strange architecture of the empty days. My throat tightened with the imagined lump of globus hystericus. I heard the bin men come and go in the morning, and would sit and try to write, listening to the hum of the fridge in the deserted house. I made elaborate dinners and watched the same TV headlines at one and six. Something would come up, I told myself. It always did.

After months of creeping anxiety, I had to say something. I

hadn't known how to tell her how I was feeling, as we lay curled against each other on the sofa – so I had kept quiet. I was terrified that nothing would work out, and as the weeks passed it had begun to feel like a charade, hiding my doubts and anxiety until I couldn't do it any more. Breaking up seemed like the easiest option. At least then I wouldn't have to explain. I could slip back into the safety of silence.

'I'm sorry,' I said, aware of the water lapping at my feet, 'it just doesn't feel right.'

'What now, then?' she replied, her voice breaking. 'Do we go home together to *our* house?'

I was aware of both the time and distance that separated us from the shore. I needed to say something to make it stop.

'Is it about sex?' she asked, as the boat glided between strokes.

'Yes – no – I don't know.'

I wanted to tell her how hard I found it to slip down into my body and suggest how to be touched, or to explore what for so many years was forbidden, as I felt the soft weight of her breasts in bed. But I had never made peace with sex. Instead, without saying anything, I had withdrawn, until my body was physically clenched like a clam. Fear, sex and silence: for me it always came back to this trinity.

'I'm so sorry.'

The boat docked. The man at the pier said something about 'smiling, as it might never happen' – and I wanted to hit him. We passed him the foam husks we had been wearing in silence, and she walked away without speaking. I watched the dark outline of her retreating footprints, as they vanished in the sun.

I tried to catch her hand. 'Please,' I said, 'I'm sorry. I don't know what I want. I just didn't know how to talk to you. I don't want this to end. But I don't know what else to do. Please.'

'Why?' she said, inscrutable behind her sunglasses. 'Why do you find it so hard to tell me what's going on?

And I knew. I knew I had to tell her if we were to survive. I had to explain why I struggled to say what I felt – and how I buried feelings so deep that I hadn't been able to express even my most basic sexual needs until I was in my thirties. Slowly, carefully, I explained about the boot room, and the Volvo and the unheated house. The quotidian tragedies that were enough to quieten me. I suggested that somehow these silences had seeped into my life – and that they were part of why I couldn't explain how I felt, or articulate my doubts. And why that pull was always there, dragging me back to silence and separation. Where it was safer.

'Well, you've got to figure this stuff out,' she said, turning away, 'or this will never work.'

She was right. Silence had somehow become tangled up with sex – the meeting of bodies where there are no words – and it is only now that I am beginning to unpick it. It has always been in sexual relationships that I have struggled to say what I mean. I have friendships that have lasted a lifetime – but it is this most intimate form of communication that has eluded me.

Now more than ever, I need to know why.

TRIG POINT

I CAME TO SEX LATE in life. At school it was a source of constant shame that I had only ever kissed a boy – never anything more. The autumn term began with a terrible ritual known as 'corruption'. The older girls would sit on your bed and ask you what certain terms meant – a 'pearl necklace' or a 'golden shower' – as the rest of the dormitory looked on. Sometimes the questions were more physical, and you might be asked to perform a blow-job on a can of Impulse body spray. I was terrified – as I knew almost nothing. I was in my twenties when I finally had sex for the first time. And the fact that I came to sex late meant it often seemed strangely frantic, as though making up for lost time.

With my first boyfriend, we would touch each other in the pink glow of my fairy lights, holding our breath to keep the noise down in a shared student house of five girls. And as the months went on, it began to feel desperate: thrusting together in the back of a car, with face paint running into my eyes after a friend's twenty-first, or fully clothed beside a trig point on a Scottish mountain – wiping myself on the spongy moss as walkers approached.

The deep, visceral connection of sex was intoxicating, and I genuinely believed it would bind us together forever. When I moved to Berkeley, six months after we met, it just seemed like a hiccup in our star-crossed relationship. We would talk late at night, and I constructed a parallel universe, building my days around the calls to him – trying to use a webcam in the shared computer lab and writing letters for the first time in my life.

It was around this time that I first encountered George Oppen, and in the breathless throes of my own first love I saw myself mirrored in his relationship with his wife Mary. She was his touchstone, his muse – for 'when I say Love I mean Mary', he wrote in one of his posthumously published daybooks.[1] They met when Mary was a student at the University of Oregon, and George sat in the front row of her contemporary poetry classes. Mary says she 'found George Oppen and poetry at one moment'.[2]

In many ways, Mary is the keeper of George's story, for her autobiography *Meaning a Life* is the only full account of their lives together. She describes their meeting as a miracle, and remembers that for their desperately romantic first date, George collected her in his roommate's Model T Ford and they 'drove into the country, sat and talked, made love, and talked until morning' under the light of a moon that 'made such a white light we could almost see colours'.[3] George described the night, decades later, in his poem 'The Forms of Love', in which he recalls:

A lake beside us
When the moon rose.
I remember

Leaving the ancient car
Together. I remember
Standing in the white grass
Beside it. We groped
Our way together
Down-hill in the bright
Incredible light[4]

From that night on, Mary says, 'our response to each other was always to stay together',[5] with their relationship pitted against the conventional demands of the world. In the morning after their date, when Mary returned to her dormitory, she was expelled from college for staying out past curfew (while George was only suspended). And in the weeks and months that followed, the young couple turned their backs on what was expected of them and hitchhiked across the US and travelled through France, before settling in New York in the 1930s.

Visitors to the couple's Polk Street apartment in San Francisco some fifty years later would recall George and Mary still moving in each other's orbit like the needles of a compass: 'turning upon a single, unseen centre',[6] and always speaking in the first-person plural. Young writers flocked to join their coterie, and many have written about simply enjoying being in their presence. As

Mary recalled, 'The young people now come to visit, to talk and they seem happy to look at us, survivors. Perhaps they are strengthened by a view of us which represents fifty years together in a fully lived life. This achievement, be it luck or choice, has been inevitable.'[7]

HAIR

DURING MY TIME AT BERKELEY I was cast in *The Vagina Monologues*. I was trying to make friends beyond the cooperative and had got involved in student drama, as I had always found other people's words easier to say – like the poetry that had tripped me out of silence, years before. But something about this play floored me. I simply couldn't do it. I remember sitting in the computer lab when they sent me my script, unable to imagine how I would say the words out loud. The communal printer sat squat at the opposite end of the room and I knew I could not even print the script. The show was to be performed on Valentine's Day, and I was the first onstage. The title of the monologue: 'Hair'.

Absurdly, my boyfriend and I called my vagina the naughty place; the words fraught with childish shame. The monologue itself echoes this complicated relationship with sex. It is about a woman whose husband wants her to shave her vagina, leaving it 'puffy and exposed and like a little girl' because 'this excited him'.[8] As the first monologue of the show, it is rich with one-liners: 'You have to love hair in order to love the vagina', Eve Ensler writes, as it is the 'leaf around the flower'.[9] But the piece has a darker edge. The husband leaves and 'screws around' because his wife won't shave her cunt. And the couple end up in marital therapy, with the wife blamed for his infidelity. In hindsight, it's a powerful polemic about male power and how it trumps female desire, but at the time I couldn't see any of this. I just knew I couldn't stand on stage and say the word 'vagina'. And so I replied to the email, and made my apologies; I was too busy for feminism that year.

It is one of the very few things in my life that I have turned down. I have travelled to Afghanistan and Iraq, where the spectacle of a woman filming on the streets was enough to stop traffic, and I have backpacked alone through South America fresh from school with only phrasebook Spanish. But something about saying the word vagina on stage was impossible. I was ashamed that I couldn't stand up and perform this feminist act. But eventually I got parts in other plays and buried thoughts of this first refusal – until events conspired to bring me back to Eve Ensler.

It was the summer of the argument in the rowing boat, and I was once again living parallel lives: travelling across the world for work, and spending every other weekend at our flat in London. I was not really present in either place. Eve was one of the interviewees for the series on women's rights that I was filming, and the week before the argument in Hyde Park I had been sitting in her apartment in Manhattan, talking about feminism. The walls were lined floor to ceiling with editions of her books, their pink spines pressed against each other. I had expected to hate her. Reading *The Vagina Monologues* on the plane, they seemed crass, obvious and a bit irrelevant: I for one have never thought about what my vagina would wear, and I couldn't see what talking about it had to do with feminism. But in person Eve was hard not to like. Newly recovered from cancer, she radiated energy and enthusiasm. She was passionate about the importance of naming the female anatomy; in bringing it from darkness into plain sight. I was too ashamed to tell her that I had been unable to perform her words, all those years ago.

For years after we met I kept thinking about her, and her belief in the importance of talking openly about sex, without shame or embarrassment. I had never said 'vagina' so many times as we did during that interview – and it was liberating. I had been able to almost feel new neural pathways being formed as we spoke the taboo. And as I began to explore my own inability to speak the truth in sexual relationships, I kept thinking back to her and that afternoon in Manhattan. I could think of no one else who has been so instrumental in breaking open the taboos about the female body and insisting that we talk openly and honestly about sex and sexuality. If anyone knows how to dispel the shame and silence around sex it is Eve Ensler. It has been her life's work for women to be able to talk about their desires openly.

And so, after several emails to her assistant, I arrange to travel halfway around the world to meet Eve again – first to New York, and then to her farm, upstate. I don't even know the address.

'Eve will meet you,' her assistant tells me. He answers all the emails I send to her, and arranges the date of our meeting. It feels a little like going to the Emerald City, hoping to see the Wizard of Oz behind the curtain.

I catch the bus from the central terminal in Manhattan, and as soon as I leave New York, it feels almost as though the city does not exist – the skyscrapers quickly giving way to broad-porch timber houses, with jack o' lanterns still grinning from Halloween.

When we meet, Eve is wearing black – leggings and a rollneck. She has bought cakes for the occasion – far more than two people could or should eat at one sitting – and presses them into my hand in a ziplock bag for the bus journey back. She is sweet, concerned and smaller than I remember when she meets me at the bus stop, perched at the wheel of an enormous four by four. On the drive from the bus station, she talks about me, asking about my writing and why I have become so interested in why words sometimes desert us. So I tell her about getting married, and the gaping silences of the boot room, and my growing interest in the sexually unspeakable. For someone who has made their name talking about themselves, it is strangely hard to divert the conversation back to her.

Her kitchen looks out onto a pond and an impenetrable dark wood. Coming here feels like being let in on a secret; the location is not advertised online, and it is a shift from the confessional disclosure that made her name.

It is dark by the time we start talking, and the night lends the conversation a certain intimacy. I turn on the dictaphone, and she pours more tea. There is something incongruous about the finger cakes and cookies and our conversation.

'So tell me,' I say, 'do you remember when you first said the word "vagina"?'

Eve first performed *The Vagina Monologues* in a café, moving quickly to Here, which she describes as a 'tiny theatre in downtown New York'.[10] When later I tried to find Here, as part of my pilgrimage to Eve's farm, I walked straight past. The road opposite was being ripped apart by construction work, and people hurried by to try and escape the bitter New York winter. There was a smart ski store, and a Middle Eastern boutique opposite, which distracted my attention. And when I eventually found the entrance, it was closed. There was no sense that this place was important in the history of pushing the boundaries of what we can and cannot say. But it was.

Eve recalls that, at the point she walked onto that stage for the opening night in 1996, you couldn't say 'vagina' in a gynaecologist's office, let alone in public.[11] It was the 'naughty place' or, as one woman puts it, in the *Monologues*, her 'pussy cat'. The list of euphemisms Eve collected when researching the show is seemingly endless, such was the taboo around female genitalia.

Famously, the show grew from a discussion about the menopause, which shocked Eve as she had never heard the vagina talked about with such contempt – as something 'dried up' and useless. This led her to conduct over 200 interviews with women about their vaginas, primarily because she was 'curious'. But she was worried about the reception her curiosity would receive. 'I honestly thought I would be shot,' she laughs, recalling the opening night. 'It was utterly terrifying, and I was scared for a long time, with every different audience, you know? But I was also excited. It's that moment when you're about to break through something, a taboo or a wall, and it's terrifying and exciting all at the same time.'

The monologues chart most areas of female sexual experience, from first orgasms to pubic hair, sexual harassment, birth, and rape in the course of war. Reading early reviews of the show, it sounds as though she was right to worry about its reception. James Langton in the *Daily Telegraph* wrote that the show was 'more euphemistically known in some quarters, simply as the monologues',[12] and even as late as 2007, one production in Florida was renamed the *HooHaa Monologues*, for fear of causing offence. The news report I read said Eve didn't approve.[13] Because, of course, cutting the word 'vagina' from the title completely misses the point. The monologues only have meaning because they name and reclaim the female body. They speak the unsayable.

Eve is passionate about why it matters to say the word 'vagina', likening it to a divine act – calling the body into being by naming it. 'Talking about your vagina gives you agency over it,' she says, 'it makes it real, makes it concrete.' Female sexuality, she says, has been shrouded in shame 'since Eden', and naming the female body, in public, can go some way to erasing that shame. Once women talk openly about their sexual experiences, be that orgasms, short skirts or harassment, 'it creates a community' and a recognition of a shared experience, which can be empowering. 'You know, I keep thinking it will become irrelevant,' she continues, 'and every year I say to my team, "Well, I guess this is the last year", but the truth of the matter is it's oddly more relevant now than it's ever been. Places are signing up to do it this year because they *have to*, not because it's a reminiscence, or some kind of nostalgia piece.' She goes on, 'I think we are still in a place where women don't know what their bodies are or what they like sexually, what pleasures them – and I still don't think women are able to tell men that.' And the net result is that 'I think men don't even know to a certain degree what sexual harassment is, or what consent means.'

It would be easy to mock Eve and the idea of making your vagina 'real' – but we are talking at a strange time. When we meet at her farm, it is at the height of the #metoo movement, and hundreds of thousands of women across the world have begun to tell their stories of sexual abuse and violation, in the wake of allegations against Hollywood producer Harvey Weinstein. In the weeks that follow, *Time* magazine names the 'Silence Breakers' its 'people of the year'. It feels as though the act of telling your story – moving the female body out of the darkness and into plain sight – is in the very air. And this talking and telling was, in many ways, prefigured by *The Vagina Monologues*. 'This is fifty years of work coming to be,' Eve says, 'and then there's this zeitgeist moment where it all goes boom.' She stops and looks directly across the kitchen table at me. 'What we don't talk about doesn't exist – and what happens to vaginas happens in the dark, and in silence. If you don't talk about it, you don't know it's ever happened. Breaking the silence is critical – it saves your life. If you break the silence it frees you.'

Eve is talking from deeply personal experience. For much of her adult life she harboured a secret, which, like all secrets, began to insidiously infect everything it touched. It drove her halfway around the world, and to the edge of obliteration through drink and drugs in her twenties. 'I was living in the darkness and secrecy of that story,' Eve says. 'It was always spinning in my head. I was always blaming myself, I just felt sick. I felt sick from it, literally.'

The secret she harboured was this: from the ages of five to ten Eve was repeatedly raped by her father, who then became physically abusive, until she was able to leave the family home as a teenager. From the outside, you would not have known what was happening, as she writes in her memoir *Insecure at Last*: 'I grew up in a middle-class family and neighbourhood in the United States. I had plenty of food, clothes. I had my teeth straightened. I took ballet classes. We went on vacations.'[14] But this came at a price: 'My father was a raging alcoholic. His anger permeated and infected my world. His fists, his hand, his belts, marked my young body and my being.'[15]

From the beginning, the abuse was marked by a strange double-think, a denial of reality by everyone around Eve. She would come down to breakfast in the morning, and her father would ask where she got the bruises on her neck – from his stranglehold the night before. There was a conspiracy of silence. Everyone knew, but did not know. And so she learnt not to tell. To wait. She writes in her memoir that she would sit on the front porch waiting for someone to rescue her.

She says her mother could not process the truth of what was

going on, even years after the event. 'I mean, look,' Eve says, 'she knew what was happening. All the signs were there; I would scream in my bed night after night. But my mother was a poor woman who married a rich man, and she had three kids – where was she gonna go? I understand it all on a certain level. But on another level . . .' There simply are no words.

CONSPIRACY OF SILENCE

EVE LEAVES ME AT THE bus stop, and I sit, pulling my coat around me against the cold, thinking back to our conversation. It was hard to know what to say – how to meet her matter-of-fact description of abuse and incest. 'Sorry' feels totally inadequate. When I play the recording of the conversation back, weeks later, I cringe at my clumsy silences, as I fumbled for the next question. I felt ill-equipped to talk about these terrible sexual experiences with her. The strange thing about sex for me is that for most of my adult life it has been totally absent – for after my eventual, joyful, discovery of sex, it became taboo.

My ex-boyfriend and I stopped having sex a few months before the relationship finally ran its course. In hindsight, the withdrawal of physical intimacy helped create space when we couldn't find the words to say 'This is over'. But it didn't just peter out; in a stab of conscience, he decided we should stop sleeping together, saying we should instead reconsecrate sex for marriage. Rather than simply breaking up, physical intimacy was reframed as something that could start again later – omnipresent but perennially deferred. And so sex was broken down into its component parts; there could be touching, but not penetration.

And so, the silly spontaneity of those early days was replaced by puritanical shame. Shame for my ongoing desire, and shame for the fact we couldn't make it work. If only we could love each other enough for a lifetime commitment, he said, then sex could start again – an absurd, unobtainable prize. Looking back, I don't know why I didn't leave. I thought it was love, I suppose. It was such a brief liaison in many ways; no more than a few years on the brink of adulthood – but the shame of the withdrawal of sex stayed with me. By stopping sleeping together, we had put sex back into the shackles of age-old Christianity, puritanical shame and masculine power. With hindsight, that sexual withdrawal shaped what I would become for the next ten years of my life: closed, scared and bent out of shape by the shameful secret that I was not desirable enough, and unable to trust my body.

What strikes me now is that I didn't say anything. Or rather, I did – we fought and I shouted and I pleaded – and none of it made any difference. I remember running down the central artery of the city and scratching the back of my own hands in frustration. It is the closest I have ever come to self-harm. My language didn't work. Nothing changed, no matter what I said. He had decided and that was that. So much of sex is about power – whether it is forcing it on someone, or withdrawing it. To me that's the heart of #metoo – it's not about misplaced desire, it's about power. The power to reach into someone else's world, their space, their body, without permission. And to leave without apology.

After my boyfriend and I broke up, I withdrew from sex for almost a decade. There was the occasional kiss at a party, but never more than that. I became celibate, unable to reach out to people physically. Those early sexual experiences encased me in another layer of silence: I didn't know how to start forming relationships with other people after this first romance had gone so disastrously wrong, and I couldn't explain how I had become so seemingly unlovable.

*

I began to look for patterns – to try to see how other people's early sexual experiences shaped who they became. All I knew of Oppen's sexual experience was his well-documented relationship with Mary. But what came before? I find the answer in an excerpt from his daybooks, which were published in an avant-garde literary journal in the 1980s. I can hardly believe what I am reading: Oppen's first sexual experiences were with his step-mother.

He writes about it only once, and the language is fractured and elliptical, as though he can't quite bring himself to say the words. His early years in New Rochelle were happy enough, but after his mother's death, when he was seven, his father remarried and the family moved across the country to the west coast of America. It was, Mary says in a later interview, a wrench for George. And there, in San Francisco, the shape of the family was recast, with Oppen pitted directly against his stepmother. Describing this time, he writes, 'with my father's second marriage there opened on me an attack totally murderous, totally brutal, involving sexual attack, beatings'. And so he 'set [himself] to survive', even though he didn't think '[his] chances very good'.[16]

As for Eve, the beatings were in plain sight, and yet unspoken, as they were 'disguised by the assistance of doctors', and even though Oppen writes that he 'responded classically' with 'bed-wetting, a terrifying asthma attack', these signs were also denied and dismissed as hysterical symptoms. 'The asthma attack', he writes, was 'misdefined (as is for some reason typical in my family) as a mysterious ailment called paralysed throat'.[17] Reading this, I can't help but think of Blanche, the hysterical queen of the Salpêtrière Hospital, who had also been molested in her youth and whose throat would close in physical spasms of unspeakable distress.

Oppen summarises the situation heartbreakingly, stumbling through compound parentheses to find the words: '(sexual: unable to believe the . . . or even / complicity of an adult woman (and my father's wife) I assumed all guilt (of thought, of reaction) was mine) (age 12)'.[18] It seems to me that the grown man was still not quite able to recount the experience openly, even as a private diary entry, and had to keep the confession in closed brackets. The experience is only mentioned once in the excerpts from the daybooks; it is a footnote, almost. I feel strange dragging it centre-stage. It seems too painful, too private. And yet it is important. For this secret somehow distorted the world around it for Oppen.

As for Eve, the secret abuse and misplaced guilt bent Oppen's early life out of shape – and whereas in the 1960s Eve sought out sex and drugs, Oppen writes that the secret abuse drove him to 'suicidal driving and game playing, fist fighting, the acceptance of any dare at all'[19] as life seemed increasingly worthless. Six weeks before he was due to graduate from high school, Oppen was the driver in a serious accident in which a man was killed. He was expelled from school for drinking and his life took a very different course – one which would eventually lead him to Oregon and to Mary.

It is interesting that the boy whose beatings were disguised by doctors would come to write poetry that insists – above all else – that we *see what is really going on*. Or, as he writes in 'Route':

> Clarity, clarity, surely clarity is the most beautiful
> > Thing in the world,
> A limited, limiting clarity.[20]

Oppen writes time and again that his poetry must be 'honest', 'sincere', as the poem's only real function is to communicate faithfully the truth about the world. Perhaps this is because, as a child, he was 'unable to believe' what was being done to him by his 'father's wife'.

But even in his insistence on 'clarity' there is more going on. To me, the space before 'Thing in the world' suggests something unsaid, a caesura, a physical pause on the page, which he cannot find the words to fill. Perhaps this is because, as he writes in 'Of

Being Numerous', 'the known and unknown / Touch'[21] and everything we see suggests something beyond our sight; the gap between recognising the symptoms of a 'paralysed throat' and spotting the signs of abuse perhaps.

Just as Oppen's poetry privileges the act of seeing, so Eve's drama foregrounds listening and telling – perhaps as a reaction to the unspeakable secrets she carried through adolescence.

Back at her kitchen table in upstate New York, Eve tells me that this impulse to listen to and recount other people's stories began as a young activist, when she worked in a women's shelter. The fact that no one believed her own story – even in the face of physical bruising from the beatings – meant that she wanted to bear witness to the abuse suffered by others. 'I wanted to show up for people,' she says. 'I wanted to hear them, I wanted to cry with them, I wanted to let them know I felt what they are feeling.' This quest led her across the globe, from women's shelters in New York to Bosnia, Pakistan and Afghanistan, where she was almost whipped by the Taliban. She sneaked across borders and sweated in refugee camps with scant regard for her own safety or well-being. 'It was about wanting to be a witness,' she says, 'wanting to hear other people – to give what I needed the most.'

In many ways, *The Vagina Monologues* was the greatest act of listening. 'I didn't know what I thought about my vagina,' Eve says, 'and I didn't know what other women thought about their vaginas, so it was really curiosity, and then the deeper in I got the more amazed and horrified and excited I was by what women were saying – and I kept following it because it was compelling.'

But once the play opened, Eve realised that by bringing vaginas out of the dark, she had created a space for women to tell stories they had never been able to articulate before. 'What was really exciting was to see the response,' she says, 'and how immediate it was; how after every single show women lined up to talk to me.' She leans across the table, theatrically. 'They said they *had to* tell me their stories – they had to – so I would just sit there, listening and listening, and sometimes I would invite people over to my apartment and I would spend hours with women, and sometimes I would just sit and listen, as I just knew these women *needed to tell their story.*'

Eve had unearthed a well of unspoken sexual abuse. By breaking the taboo around the word 'vagina', she had somehow given women permission to talk about the unspeakable things that had been done to them. And so, night after night, they came and spoke to her – of the rapes, incest, harassment and shame. 'I did not know the show would be a catalyst for that kind of storytelling,' she says. 'I had no idea. I mean, I knew there were women who had been violated, obviously, I was violated, but I had no idea of the epic proportions.' And so, after reclaiming the word 'cunt' onstage, Eve would listen to stories of abuse. The stories she had never been able to tell.

But telling was not enough. From the very beginning of *The Vagina Monologues*, Eve had a deep sense of responsibility for the women whose stories she had become custodian of – and an awareness of a growing community who had survived horrendous physical and sexual abuse. 'It was a real honour,' she says. 'I felt it was a privilege to be the receiver of those stories.' But the sheer scale of the abuse required something alongside the storytelling. The silence had been broken. The next question was what to do about it.

As Eve recalls, she gathered a group of women in her apartment a few years after the first performance and said that they needed to find a way to use the *Monologues* to raise awareness about sexual violence, and abuse, towards women and girls – so that Eve was not just 'a war photographer', but was part of the solution. 'I couldn't just take those stories, and do nothing,' she says. 'I felt an incredible sense of responsibility.' Since then, the *Monologues* have been performed every year on Valentine's Day, for free, with the profits going to local charities. The performances are part of V-Day – with the V standing for victory, Valentine, and of course vagina.[22] Gala V-Day performances were embraced by the Hollywood elite: Susan Sarandon, Whoopi Goldberg, Kate Winslet, Jane Fonda, the list goes on. The first V-Day performance in New York's Hammerstein ballroom raised $250,000 in one night,[23] and in 2001 V-Day sold out at Madison Square Gardens, raising $1 million. It was a V-Day performance that I would have taken part in in Berkeley in 2004 – and in 2018, V-Day celebrated its twentieth anniversary. But beside the pink feather boas, and star value, Eve was also confronting her own story.

She is unsure when exactly she told her mother about the abuse – but tells me it was sometime during this period of *The Vagina Monologues*. 'It was really hard,' she says, 'it was really scary; you feel like the whole world is going to tumble down; you feel like all the walls of the house are going to collapse.

You feel you will be left and abandoned, and people aren't going to believe you . . . and people will think you're dirty, and you'll be humiliated, and it's horrible. But I did know as a storyteller that stories are liberation.' She pauses. 'Look, the moment I told my mother what my father had done to me was the hardest thing I've ever done – but a depression I had carried my entire life lifted in that moment. It was gone. I was no longer depressed. It was over and it's never come back.'

In another interview, Eve has said that she didn't tell her mother to get sympathy or to hear that she was loved – but just to say, 'this happened, and you need to know'.[24] Listening to her speak, I am reminded of an Oppen poem, in which he describes the value of telling, for it is all we are ever able to do:

> I might at the top of my ability stand at a window
> And say, look out; out there is the world.
> Not the desire for approval nor even for love – O,
> That trap![25]

It seems to me he is talking about exactly what Eve experienced; to tell without thought of acceptance or hope of love.

CAN I HELP YOU?

IN THE DAYS AND WEEKS after the end of that first sexual relationship at university, I lost the plot. I moved to London and started training as a journalist. I would walk out of lectures into the snow, or sit on buses long past my stop. The year before we broke up, my boyfriend had made a wax maquette of a couple for me, twisted together in a ball. The wax figures were temporary, he said, intended to be fired off in the kiln. He said he would cast it in bronze for our first anniversary, if we got married – once sex was clean and worthwhile again. I gave it back to him the following year, cradled in a plastic bag. I was living in a tiny flat which had mites on the bathroom walls. The garden was a tangle of brambles that had grown around an abandoned car, where foxes would sun themselves in the brisk December afternoons. The flat didn't have a living room, so my life felt as though it had collapsed physically, folding itself into the four walls of my bedroom.

I threw myself into work, and, looking back, I recognise something of Eve in myself – in going to the ends of the world to hear other people's stories. This was a time at which I said 'yes' to everything professionally. I went to Afghanistan – four times in five years. I remember the week before my first trip, on the hostile-environment training course, we had to run into a simulated terror attack. I stumbled into a basement, in the dark, with the sound of gunfire played on a loop, looking for actors playing wounded journalists and civilians, my fingers sticky with fake blood. I learnt how to treat a sucking chest wound, and how to make a stretcher out of three coats. Everyone else laughed it off with drinks in the bar that evening, but I was really shaken. Somewhere a voice was asking, 'Why are you doing this?' I wanted someone to notice. To ask if I was OK.

My first job, the year after we broke up, was working shifts for a news agency – going to court and watching other people's lives fall apart, and driving through the night to get to train crashes. The hours were shift-based, and I found myself with time on my hands. I would watch mid-morning television, with ad breaks for hearing aids and Mediterranean cruises, and then miss nights out because I was staying at the office. I needed something to fill the empty hours when my shifts didn't line up with everyone else, and I had time to think. I saw an advert for Samaritans in the local paper one morning. They needed volunteers, particularly people who could help out during the day or late at night – the times when the silence and loneliness were at their worst. I went along to an information morning.

Thinking back to that time, I am reminded of Eve's edict that you should 'give what you need the most'. In those narrow lonely days I needed compassion. I cringe re-reading emails to my ex sent that winter: the anger smarting on the page. I needed help to meet the deep sadness of not being able to control what was happening. Not being able to be loved enough, or listen to his explanations, and sending email after email but never getting the salve I needed in return.

In some ways, Samaritans enabled me to give what I needed the most in that first single year: compassion, time and attention. And it taught me for the first time in my life what real communication looked like. How to listen, and how to be heard.

As new volunteers, we were taught that the aim was to listen to people without judging, or offering advice. I remember on the first day of training we did an exercise with a man dressed as a washing machine. The idea was that he would play the role of caller and we could experiment with being the 'Samaritan', as we went around the circle. It became immediately clear that his washing machine had broken – and as novices we tried to offer solutions: 'Have you thought of calling a plumber?' or 'Could you use the local launderette?' But these attempts at problem-solving led nowhere and made him retreat further behind the cardboard carapace.

It was only when the more experienced Samaritans suggested asking how he was coping, or what was the hardest thing about the lack of a washing machine, that he started to emerge, and we heard about a life of chronic isolation, bereavement and disgust at himself for not being able to solve this simple problem. He talked about self-harm and fleeting suicidal thoughts. I had never heard a conversation like this. It felt as though the world was opening up. Here, finally, was a guide to how to speak with other people. In the weeks to come we were equipped with the tools to listen, which taught us that we could reflect or summarise what was being said, look for more information, or clarification, or simply offer sounds of encouragement. The emphasis was on being a human being, finding the words that felt natural to you and keeping it conversational. And yet this was so different to the way most conversations – or rather *my* conversations – developed. Rather than nudging someone towards what you are comfortable with, and telling them to 'pull themselves together', we were encouraged to go with them into the silence unfolding.

I remember sitting in the dead of night listening to people telling me unspeakable things that they couldn't tell anyone else, for fear of being sectioned or simply not heard. I loved that I was not expected to offer opinions or answers. Very often we would just sit in silence. And yet, the founding principle of Samaritans is that you cannot and will not tell anyone else what is said on the phone – so I cannot write about the calls I have taken, or the calls other volunteers have told me about. Once again I am circling silence; like trying to talk to the selective mutes, as part of my research, who would only reply via email.

In desperation I start looking for callers who have shared their stories, and I come across a woman called Sophie, who was in contact with Samaritans throughout the 1980s and documented her experiences in her autobiography, *Scarred*. She first called Samaritans from a phone box, at the point at which her life had become unbearable. She was fourteen and had been sexually abused by her adoptive father from the age of twelve.

He would rape her, before inviting friends to come and gang-rape her in her childhood bedroom. She coped by self-harming, but once he saw her cutting herself he began to join in – stubbing out cigarettes on her and commenting on how she enjoyed pain. She recounts in graphic detail how she tried to end her life on several occasions, once when she found out she was pregnant with her father's child at the age of fifteen. She had already become pregnant by him once before, and knew she could not go through with another abortion, and so spun the authorities a story about her 'boyfriend'. Her life was a 'spiral of suicidality' from which she saw no escape.[26]

She writes that she is in no doubt that it was Samaritans who saved her life. She first called them after a night of particularly horrendous abuse. From then on she was 'befriended' by two Samaritans volunteers, who were in contact with her throughout her adolescence. In an interview with the BBC World Service, Sophie explained that it was the confidentiality Samaritans offered that allowed her to treat them as a 'safe place' where she could explain things she could not tell anyone else. It was, she says, essential that she knew no one was going to 'swoop in' and save her – or take her away from her father. He had drilled into her that as she had been adopted he was all she had in the world, and the thought of losing him or disappointing him was almost worse than the abuse. And so it was only knowing that her contact with Samaritans was confidential that allowed her to talk honestly about what was happening to her, and about her feelings of despair, without having to worry that social services would get involved and take her away.[27]

It seems counter-intuitive that Sophie would have wanted to stay with her father – but through their policy of being non-judgemental and confidential, Samaritans became a source of support when all else had failed. Sophie was eventually sent to a secure mental institution for her own safety, as she was a risk to herself, and from there began the painstaking process of recovery. Such was her gratitude to Samaritans that she went on to become a volunteer, branch leader and eventually chair of the organisation from 2008 to 2011.

Like Sophie, I knew that Samaritans was different from any other organisation, with their emphasis on confidentiality and non-judgemental listening without the need to find answers. I had had conversations and heard things I would not have thought possible, and I was amazed that by simply not offering solutions people could be helped to speak more. In many ways I wished I had called them when I was younger. As I was training to be a volunteer, I would occasionally ring them, during low moments, and listen to the voice on the end of the phone saying, 'Samaritans, can I help you?' I never said anything back. Sitting in silence with someone for a few minutes was enough.

UNCONSECRATED GROUND

I AM SITTING IN THE basement of the BFI film archives, just off Tottenham Court Road. The room is empty apart from three old television sets, a stack of VHS cassettes, and a plate of digestive biscuits. I play the first tape. It opens in Lincoln, with a vicar walking slowly around a graveyard in a long black cassock. As he walks, he tells the story of how as a young man he was called to conduct the funeral of a child. It was a last-minute substitution, and he arrived late, knowing nothing about the child that had died. He was told by the undertaker that she had taken her own life. As a result, the funeral party were forced to walk across the open fields to a plot of unconsecrated ground for the burial. It was the 1930s and suicide was illegal, so she could not be buried in the churchyard. By a strange quirk of fate, the undertaker's own daughter had been at school with the dead girl, and said that she had apparently taken her own life when she had started her period. The rush of blood was terrifying to her, and she thought she was dying.[28]

It started to rain as they began the burial. The undertakers wore potato sacks over their heads to keep dry and the mourners quickly left the graveside to get under cover. The vicar stood alone at the side of the grave and spoke to the corpse: 'Little girl,' he said, 'I never knew you, but you have changed my life. I promise you that I will teach children your age what they need to know, and be someone they can ask, even if I get called a dirty old man at the age of twenty-four.'[29]

The experience of burying the little body in unconsecrated ground stayed with the vicar, and he spent his life trying to make sure that shame, or embarrassment, about sex would not drive anyone else to despair. In an interview shortly before his death, he said that he hoped he would be remembered as Britain's first sex therapist[30] – but he is perhaps better known as the Reverend Prebendary Chad Varah. Several decades after the little girl's funeral he would go on to found Samaritans, which was at the time the world's first telephone helpline.

I stop the tape. I had not known that the organisation was founded on horror and shame about the female body. The same gut-wrenching shame that drove Eve to perform *The Vagina Monologues* sixty years later, and that tangled me up in silence and shame throughout my twenties.

Sitting in the BFI basement, I am reminded of a filming trip through the mountains of far west Nepal – where I encountered women who were, like the little girl buried in unconsecrated ground, terrified of their own bodies. We were investigating Chhaupadi, or the taboos around menstruation. In some regions of Nepal, girls are required to sleep separately from their families when they have their periods; the women we filmed had to use a different water source while they were bleeding, and could not eat certain foods or touch certain plants or animals. They would sleep in crawlspaces under their houses, where they were vulnerable to the elements, and also to any passing men.[31] The taboos ran deep and we spoke to women who honestly believed their hands would shrivel to claws if they touched cattle while they were bleeding. The fear and ignorance around menstruation was as real there as it had been in 1930s Lincoln.

The memory of the trip has stayed with me, especially as while I was in Nepal I had my period. I began to bleed in the dank, mosquito beds of Dhangadhi by the Indian border. There were no flushing toilets in the villages, so I spent the week balling tampons into plastic bags and stuffing them into my rucksack, to throw away at the hotel. I did not want the women to know I was menstruating, as I had to break all the taboos in order to film: touching men, eating food, using the water sources. And so I became complicit somehow in the myths, by keeping my period a secret.

At the same time, I had never talked so much about menstruation as during that trip. In the West, we value discretion – adverts show towels absorbing clear blue liquid or women dancing on beaches – seemingly denying the mess and fuss of bleeding. And periods are not spoken of; we are squeamish about blood and leaks and talk in euphemisms – the curse or a visit from aunt flo. The conversations in Nepal gave me the same feeling of disorientation as when I first met Eve and talked about vaginas for an hour. By talking about periods, it felt as though we were physically breaking apart the taboo.

When Chad Varah embarked on fulfilling his promise to the little girl, he found gross ignorance about sex and bodily functions among young people. He says he started his self-appointed mission – to educate children about sex – the night after the little girl's funeral. He was overseeing the church youth club and began by teaching the children that the word 'sod' referred to anal sex, and in the weeks to come he would disabuse young boys of the notion that masturbating would make you go blind or cause you to grow hair on the palms on your hands.[32]

These classes at the youth club were followed by marriage counselling, and over the course of six years Chad discovered that many of the couples he saw were ignorant of the female body – specifically the function of the clitoris. He wrote, 'Out of each five couples only one of the men and two of the women knew enough to be sure of the woman having an orgasm.'[33] Faced with this ignorance, he told the couples he saw that the 'clitoris was a gift of God to enable them to enjoy sexual satisfaction' – and sent them on their way. I am stunned by the frank nature of these discussions, which took place twenty years before Kinsey's report on male sexuality, and were conducted by a man of the cloth.

Of course, Chad's teaching about sex was also firmly grounded within the boundaries of Christian theology, which places sex at the heart of a heterosexual marriage. He had the opportunity to put this point of view across in 1951 as a contributor to the popular magazine *Picture Post*, which was running a controversial series called 'Sex and the Citizen', which aimed to demystify sex for the common man. The introduction to the series said it would tackle the 'ordinary sex problems of ordinary people', as 'sex in all its manifestations is probably the most important aspect of human relationships' and yet is 'rarely discussed in an honest way'.[34] Chad was horrified by the series, which he found 'mealy mouthed and muddled',[35] so he asked if he could contribute a 'footnote'. The resulting article, 'A Parson Puts His Case', caused what Chad called 'a certain amount of stir', as it expressed his idea of a 'permissive society' where we 'permit adults to make their own moral decisions, and not to be told by the state, or by the Church, or by neighbours, what they should or should not do, or should or should not enjoy'.[36] Chad claimed that sex and sexual pleasure were a gift from God and that the human body should be enjoyed – provided, of course, this took place within the marriage bed, or, as he rather poetically puts it: 'We must not lie to one another by lying with one another when we cannot truthfully say with our voices what we are proclaiming with our bodies in the act of sexual intercourse: I love you with all my being; I belong wholly to you, only to you, always, it is in your delight that I find my own, and I praise God that he gave you to me and me to you and this to us.'[37]

Reading Chad's article makes me feel uneasy – not because of his vision of a 'permissive society', but because his description of sex is, for me, so inextricably woven into the sadness I felt as an undergraduate when sex was shelved by my boyfriend, moved off the table as not being right, or good enough. The idea that sex – offering yourself freely and openly to another person – can only mean anything, or be worth anything, if you are married, is an idea I have found profoundly damaging in the past. And so in many ways I am not surprised that the article generated a huge response.

Chad writes in his autobiography that an unprecedented number of people got in contact as a result of the article – 235 in all.[38] As he had trained as a scientist, and had an interest in statistical probability, he analysed the first 100 responses he received and was shocked to discover 13 per cent of the respondents were 'seriously suicidal'. In replying, he says he tried to steer them towards the family doctor, or a psychiatrist, but found that only one would consider going to see a 'head shrinker'. The other twelve appeared to be 'emotionally distressed rather than mentally ill'.[39] This discovery that 'emotional distress' could lead to suicidal feelings was a revelation to Chad. Rather than being referred to a psychiatrist, Chad found that the people who had contacted him benefited from simply being allowed to tell their stories. This first glimpse of the power of being able to speak in confidence, and without fear of recrimination, was a pivotal moment in the formation of the Samaritans, which has, perhaps, done more than any other voluntary organisation to decrease the levels of suicide and despair in the UK.

Chad Varah's daughter Felicity is now patron of the charity – responsible for continuing her father's vision. We meet in a smart London club, to discuss his legacy. She is considered in her responses, and always refers to her father as 'Chad', and only once slips into calling him 'Daddy'. Over coffee, she tells me: 'A lot of people think that when he buried that child in Lincoln that was the start of Samaritans – but that wasn't it at all. What that did trigger was an understanding of the fact that people were ignorant of their own bodies,' and that this ignorance and shame could cause profound distress. She continues: 'I think *Picture Post* opened his eyes to the suicide need.' She pauses. 'He'd always until that point seen himself as a sexual counsellor, someone who could help people with their sexual problems – so he always had people who came to him who had problems with their sexuality, and felt distressed and depressed about that – but he didn't link the two things up until later.'

Now he had glimpsed how befriending could enable someone to articulate what was troubling them, he concluded that 'suicide is an emergency, requiring immediate action' rather than a lengthy wait for psychiatric care. He decided what was needed was a 'sort of 999 for potential suicides',[40] but as a busy local vicar in Battersea, with a young family (triplet sons and a daughter) and a sideline writing comic strips for *The Eagle* magazine, it was not clear how Chad could put these thoughts into action.

The answer came in 1953, when he was asked to take over as Rector of St Stephen Walbrook, in the City of London. As the church was in the City, there weren't many people in the Sunday congregation. According to his daughter Felicity, it was 'just publicans, the Lord Mayor and his family', and so Chad was able to dedicate his time to setting up the fledgling helpline. In his autobiography he explains how he had decided he would need a memorable telephone number, and so called the operator to ask how he could get hold of the number 'Mansion House

9000'. The story goes that the operator asked him to wipe the dust from the dial so that he could tell her the number he was calling from – and 'I licked my thumb, cleaned off the centre of the dial and there it was: MAN 9000'. Chad took this as a sign from God and addressed the Almighty: 'I get the message. You had it waiting for me since the telephone was first installed. Now please stop because it's getting eerie.'[41]

Chad used his Fleet Street contacts to promote the service, which was christened 'The Samaritans' by the *Daily Mirror* in December 1953.[42] And thanks to this extensive press coverage, word spread about the new service and those in need began to visit Chad in the crypt. But the newspaper articles also brought a steady stream of volunteers, who had heard about the service and wanted to help. Initially Chad was dismissive of these do-gooders, as he 'thought their function was to fetch coffee' and 'make me sandwiches', but within the first year of running the Samaritans helpline he realised that they were equally capable of befriending callers, and by February 1954 he had passed on the bulk of the listening work to his volunteers, only reserving particularly difficult cases for himself. These volunteers would listen to callers in the crypt of St Stephen Walbrook – giving them time and space to talk about things which, in every other area of their lives, would be utterly taboo. And this was to be the hallmark of the new organisation: that it was run by and for ordinary people, as they were just as capable of careful empathetic listening as professionals.

Chad chose these volunteers on the basis of who he would want to speak to if he was in distress, and discounted those who were 'pious, preachy or prudish'. He impressed upon them that even though the helpline was run from the crypt of a church, it was not religious, and they were not allowed to say that they were going to pray for callers – as that could seem judgemental, or be anathema to the atheist or agnostic. He described this new form of counselling as 'listening therapy', or 'befriending', and believed it was 'more effective than counselling in the first instance'.[43]

Early volunteers remember running across London to sit with their sandwiches on their knees in the Monday volunteer meetings, and from these early meetings the organisation gradually grew until the first branches were set up in the early 1960s, in Edinburgh and then Liverpool. As the decade progressed, the branches began to operate as a more cohesive organisation, with the unifying code of practice and procedures drawn up at the first Samaritans conference in Cardiff in 1963. The founding vision of the organisation was that fewer people would die from suicide – and within a decade it seemed that this was working: England and Wales were the only countries in the world where suicide rates actually went down between the 1960s and 1970s[44] – perhaps thanks to the growth of Samaritans.

LIVERPOOL

I AM IN SEARCH OF living history. After days of reading interviews with Chad Varah, I want to talk to the people who first
developed the active listening practised by Samaritans. How did
they know what to say? And what were the stories they heard?
So I take the train to Liverpool, to meet the country's longest
serving Samaritan volunteer. I have been ill with flu for a fort-
night, and my head is heavy as I watch the world spin by. My
days have been punctuated by naps and pauses where I lose the
thread of thought. I am worried about the interview and whether
I will be able to navigate the volunteer's fifty years of experience
within an hour and a half. But it is more than that. Over the
past few days I have become aware of a nagging, all-too-familiar
anxiety about what I am doing. As I write about my ex-boyfriend
and my family, I am becoming increasingly tense. As a journalist
and Samaritan volunteer I have learnt to keep confidences, and
writing about these experiences feels like a betrayal. I don't want
to break their secrets. I am worried about the exposure of talking
openly about my life, and can hear my mother's words as she

stood in the kitchen and told me that blood ran thicker than water. There is something shameful in speaking about private lives. But I don't know if that is true any more. How many times have I told a nervous interviewee that it is important to stand up and tell your story, to bear witness to all that has happened? And yet it feels very different now that it is me.

I have been reading George Oppen on the train. In his daybooks, especially towards the end of his life, Oppen wrote that the only point of reference he trusted was his own experience. When he was taken into a nursing home with advanced Alzheimer's, pinned above his desk was a scrap of paper on which he had written that there is 'no narrative but ourselves'.[45] I love this idea – that all of life is inevitably refracted through our personal experience. Perhaps I am just making it explicit. And retelling my story can be a way of understanding something more far-reaching about the world. It cannot just be narcissism. I hope.

The door to the Liverpool branch is never closed. It is physically chained open, in a symbolic gesture to callers, and I am greeted on the threshold by a sprightly old man carrying a slightly blackened banana and a homemade mince pie. Wiping the drizzle from his glasses, he shows me around the centre and takes me into the basement, to a lime-green meeting room named in his honour.

'It's all very embarrassing,' he says, 'but I suppose I have been here a long time.'

Alan helped to set up the Liverpool branch in 1960, and has been listening at the centre ever since. He is keen to play down his five decades of service, which led to him being awarded an MBE in 2017 – and leads me swiftly up the stairs to meet the volunteers on the phones and offer me tea and cake. But if anyone knows how to coax the unspeakable from a caller it is Alan.

He tells me that the idea of the Liverpool branch came about after the former rector of the parish church died suddenly, and the congregation were then left to process their grief alone, until the new rector suggested they establish a Samaritans branch to help meet the needs of the community.

Initially, Alan says, they 'had no idea what we were doing; we none of us had a clue whether anybody was going to ring, whether we were going to be able to cope with it, whether it was going to be upsetting, whether it was going to make us angry – nothing at all'.

The phones were manned during the day by the priests in the local church, and at night volunteers, drawn from the congregation, would take over, sleeping on camp beds and waiting for the phones to ring. Night duties were in the crypt, started at eight in the evening and went on until half-past seven the following morning, at which point they would often be woken up by the buses rattling past the windows. In those days, Alan says, night duties were often spent asleep as there were so few calls. 'The thing that was disillusioning was how slow it was to grow. You know, nobody knew about it and there was no fashion for ringing agencies at that time. You need to remember, this was 1960 – there were no social work departments, and psychiatric services were very thin.'

In those early days, he says, the organisation 'struggled', as there was no support from London and no blueprint for how to train volunteers in the new art of 'befriending'. He tells me the founders of the Liverpool branch were therefore on the lookout for ideas and became very drawn to the work of Frank Lake, a priest and psychiatrist who 'had a very strange theory that personality types were acquired partly during the birth process, or certainly by the time the child was on its feet'. The theory was that 'if things went wrong at the birth, or if the child was left too long wanting food, then it developed certain psychological attitudes', and the job of the volunteers was to use these theories to understand the 'types of callers we might meet'.[46]

But once Alan started meeting callers, he found that their problems were not so much down to abstruse 'personality types' as to the day-to-day trials of living. At a time when homosexuality, abortion and suicide were all illegal, he says he spoke to many gay men who were being blackmailed about their sexuality, or desperate women trapped in loveless marriages. They would, he remembers, assist girls who had 'come over from Ireland' to get help from a local abortion clinic. But despite the breadth of problems he encountered, he began to realise that there was something fundamental that was causing all this distress – the loneliness within intimate human relationships. For many callers, Alan says, there was 'a sense of loneliness, a schism within the relationship that left people without anybody to listen to them. For most callers it was not having anybody to talk to, who had the time and the patience and tolerance to listen to what was going on.'

Alan had glimpsed this in his own parents' relationship. He remembers his mother was 'desperately unhappy' in a marriage 'which left her overworked, unfulfilled and distant'. He tells me how his father would sit in his chair smoking his pipe, and that his mother 'used to hammer on his chest, just to get him to react'. The family lived in Yorkshire, near a water-powered mill and two large reservoirs, and he recalls, 'They would quarrel frequently and she would go out and say "I'm going to throw myself in the dam". As a kid I used to think she wouldn't come back, but then,' he goes on, 'you would hear her knocking at the door at three o'clock in the morning.' It was, he says, this sense of the isolation that gnaws at the heart of the most intimate relationships which gave him a feeling for the importance of Samaritan work.

The difficulty, according to Alan, was learning *how* to listen – and how to teach the other new recruits to support callers. 'It's a very difficult thing to teach,' he says, 'and I'm not sure if we're very good at it, even now.' He says the crucial thing is to focus on what's not being said, alongside the words they are using – and to stop yourself from giving advice. 'It's as though the caller was talking to a kind of benevolent darkness, isn't it?' He says, 'It must be really agonising to pick up that telephone and ring Samaritans because, what are you putting your trust in? You know, what are you going to empty yourself into? And if you're not listening, you can't do anything for anybody.'

Before I leave, Alan shows me the first logbooks. They chart the early years of calls and visits to the Liverpool branch – in scrawling, sun-faded handwriting. I smile at the records of the first night shifts: 'Not a sausage'. Looking through them, what's remarkable is that they could be from this year, charting broken relationships, debt, loneliness, all the things that drive people to the edge of endurance.

Hearing Alan talk about his parents' marriage, and the loneliness within personal relationships, I am reminded again of Oppen. For, despite their fabled intimacy, Mary could not explain the deepest and most elemental of her experiences to her husband George. Her life was split open by sadness about the death of her children and the trauma of giving birth – and yet somehow she never found the words to tell him. Reading her autobiography, I wonder if she told him later in life, or if he was simply lost to his work. Once he started writing again, he would work for hours at a stretch and kept up a rich correspondence with friends and editors. The bulk of his letters are about his poetry – and I wonder what sort of a husband he was. And how much space there was – aside from the work of literature – to articulate the flotsam and jetsam of life.

Mary's first miscarriage happened when she was alone. She explains that she had just turned thirty and had decided she wanted a child. She then writes, in heartbreaking detail, of the repeated stillbirths and miscarriages she suffered. There was a 'fetal death' at seven months, with no explanation; a fetus handed to her in 'a hospital pan' in the operating room; a son who died at six weeks in his cradle.[47] And these traumas were unspoken – uncommunicated to Oppen – and strangely absent from his poetry, letters and daybooks.

Chronologically they also come out of nowhere in her auto-biography – never to be mentioned again. The way she opens and closes the box on this despair reminds me of some calls I have taken at Samaritans, where you ask the most anodyne question: How are you coping? Only to open a crevasse into unexpected isolation and sadness.

The greatest trauma for Mary Oppen was childbirth, perhaps because it had become so closely tied to death: 'Birth . . . I think I am afraid to write of,' she says, for 'In childbirth I was isolated; I never talked about it even to George . . . giving birth was a peak emotional experience and so entirely my own that I never tried to express it.'[48] What strikes me is that, once again, it is this acutely female and physical experience for which she can find no words – so that we are back beside the unconsecrated ground. And I am astounded that at her most vulnerable she could not find the words to tell George, the person closest to her, who she trusted the most.

But I don't want to paint a picture of Oppen as cold and unsympathetic, for as I read more about his life, I am frequently stunned by how he was able to meet the most terrible events with empathy. He is rarely seen railing against fate, rather, more often than not, he simply wishes that people could understand more of the internal torment of others. I first glimpse this attitude when reading a letter he sent to his half-sister June, shortly after discovering that his older sister Libby had apparently killed herself.

But I need to tread carefully here. For suicide can split families, and still carries a deep shame. In the notes to her Preface to Oppen's *Selected Letters*, Rachel Blau DuPlessis writes that, although Oppen believed Libby committed suicide, her death was only 'ruled a probable suicide' by the Los Angeles County Coroner, and that there are still disagreements amongst the family about how she died.

Libby was found dead in her Los Angeles apartment in January 1960, and George's letter about the event is brief:

> I think Libby must have felt of the pills simply that she would not wake up. Which is what she wanted. It was her life. No one can say that she had to grow old. It was her life. Very much her life. This happened a long time ago; from the beginning.[49]

George and Libby had a difficult relationship 'from the beginning' – she never quite fitted in with his and Mary's bohemian lifestyle. In *Meaning a Life*, Mary describes Libby as 'lost, lonely & tragic', 'a spider waiting for males', who had married straight out of school and had children 'before she had time to learn what she wanted from life'.[50] The struggles between George and Libby started when they were still young children, alone in the house with their stepmother – during the time of Oppen's bed-wetting and asthma attacks, following his stepmother's unwanted advances. Oppen felt that when he left home, he had abandoned Libby to deal with their stepmother alone, and he was wracked with guilt for much of his life. He writes after Libby's death: 'I still wake sometimes to the guilt of having deserted [her].'[51]

Of course I cannot know if, or why, Oppen's sister had taken her own life. Perhaps I have the origin myths wrong and the 'beginning' Oppen mentions is not the early abuse, but points instead to another tragedy, for before their father remarried, George and Libby's lives had already been scarred by death – as their mother Elsie had also taken her own life.

Elsie suffered a nervous breakdown when Oppen was four and Libby seven, and shot herself – later dying of the wound in hospital.[52] She is rarely mentioned in Oppen's poetry or correspondence, but in the Introduction to his *Collected Poems* he cites the death of his mother as one of his major influences. In the penultimate letter he wrote, Oppen poignantly recalls 'climbing on my mother's bed', presumably just before she died, 'and the people said to come down, and someone said let him be –'[53] His words trailing away to all the things left unsaid.

Having learnt of Libby's death, Oppen tells his younger sister June about a 'letter' from his mother – perhaps one he has just discovered in Libby's belongings – that explains the circumstances of her suicide. 'I should have seen Elsie's letter long ago,' he writes. 'No horrors either, June. Just a woman who had a nervous breakdown, and could not understand — no one then understood.' He then quotes his mother's suicide note from 1912, heartbreaking in its simplicity:

We've been happy – i love you – i worry about the children and their school and their clothes – it seems – since i did this and don't know why that I am not fitted for the business of life.

Oppen continues in his letter to June: 'That's all she said. All she could. Just, if only people then could have known – ! they just needed to know.'[54]

Re-reading this letter, I am floored by his compassion when confronted with his own mother's despair. He does not ask why she took her life, or why she worried about the children's clothes while living a life of luxury, with butlers, valets and pearls. He does not curse her for leaving him to the later unwanted advances of his stepmother, or apportion blame. He simply wishes that someone had known – for 'they just needed to know' about her suffering.

And so here is another secret that couldn't be known, couldn't be understood, woven into the history of this poet of frankness – of Open-ness, for want of a better word. And again, from this deep feeling for his mother's isolation would come a poetry that so vividly affirms our connection with each other, our joint humanity. Perhaps his recurring, urgent sense that we are all part of something greater than ourselves is a response to the terrible isolation that took his mother's life.

TELEPHONE MASTURBATORS

NOT EVERYONE WHO CALLS SAMARITANS is suicidal. We were trained in ways to talk to people about this darkest and most taboo subject, often simply echoing the kind of compassion that Oppen showed towards his own mother. But I remember on my early shifts being surprised by the number of callers who rang with a totally different end in mind: sexual gratification. When I joined, these callers were euphemistically known as TMs, or telephone masturbators, and were, we were told, simply par for the course – a certain type of man who would enjoy calling a free phone line to hear a kind female voice. The Samaritans helpline does not keep records of the levels of this type of call, but anecdotally, on some shifts – particularly the very early morning – they felt endless.

Chad Varah was aware of this type of caller – and didn't want to turn them away. From the very beginning, at the unconsecrated ground, he had placed the discussion of sexual difficulties front and centre of Samaritans' mission. And so he developed a solution that today, in the post- #metoo era, seems unthinkable.

It was called the 'Brenda line' and was developed by Chad
to give men the opportunity to discuss their sexual difficulties
and to masturbate on the phone – if that would help to alleviate
their emotional distress. Chad believed that a certain type of
female volunteer could be trained to respond to these men, and
these special volunteers were known as 'Brendas'. Although I
try to speak to former Brendas, the organisation is keen to put
this chapter of its history in the past. So the only first-hand
testimony I have is from old documentaries about the birth of
the organisation. Back in the BFI archive, one former Brenda
explains, 'There were quite a few men ringing up and saying,
can I see your knickers? Or things like what bra size are you –
and many of them didn't get much further than this. But we
decided they were obviously unhappy about something, so we
tried to think what it might be, and we decided we would set
up a special line. When these men rang on the ordinary phone
line, we would give them a special number to ring so someone
trained in dealing with sex callers could talk to them and try
and befriend them and find out what was wrong and offer some
solace.'[55]

Not everyone approved, even in the 1970s, of the Brenda
system. Alan remembers the 'Brendas' arriving in Liverpool with
disgust. 'Chad had become a menace,' he says. 'He made his
name talking about sexual difficulties to adolescents, and that
is wonderful – but it was a load of baloney trying to get it into
the Samaritans.' When asked how well the line worked, he is
equally sceptical. 'Well, they would just masturbate and then
put the phone down. I can't understand how they would get

any Samaritan experience out of it.' Perhaps because of this type of volunteer response, the Brenda line was discontinued – and as a result Chad felt that a central element of the service had been lost, and commented, 'in some places we have turned out to be less accepting of people's sexual difficulties than any other kind of difficulty.'[56]

Chad stood down as director of the London branch in 1974 to become Honorary President of Samaritans. He spent the next ten years travelling the globe, setting up the international arm of the organisation – Befrienders International – before retiring in 1986. He died twenty years later, in 2007.

Today, Samaritans has expanded its role, in an attempt to reach those most at risk of taking their own life. This work has led them into prisons, where suicide rates are considerably higher than among the general population. The Samaritans train prisoners as 'listeners', who can be called out of their cells by other prisoners to listen to their worries. The listeners are in turn supported by Samaritan volunteers who regularly visit the prison.

One former listener I spoke to said he felt 'stoically suicidal' throughout his short stay inside. Jacob Hill served an eighteen-month custodial sentence for drug-dealing at a music festival, and said suicide was an option that was always open to him. For him, the hardest things about being inside were twofold: first, there was the solitude – he spent sixteen hours a day behind his cell door; and second, it was the lack of privacy. He was fixated by the metal flap on the back of his cell door which could be opened at any point. He never knew when he would be interrupted, observed, checked on. The listeners' service seems to offer the antithesis of this: absolute confidentiality – no one can slide open the metaphorical flap. Jacob says that being a listener made his stay in prison worthwhile. He remembers walking across the yard and looking at the stars on his way to listen to a fellow prisoner, and took pride in being able to give people a moment of release. Another former listener told me that one of the most profound contacts he had was when he sat with someone for forty-five minutes while they cried. There was nothing to say, but at least they were not alone.

With the goal of reducing the number of people who commit suicide, Samaritans has also entered into partnership with Network Rail in order to prevent suicides on the railways. Dr Lisa Marzano, a psychologist at Middlesex University, told me that although only 4 to 5 per cent of suicides in the UK happen on the railways, it's an area where quick intervention can have a dramatic effect. Her research shows that many people choose the railway as they think they will not be interrupted. Samaritans has now offered listening training to hundreds of railway staff, so that they feel able to approach someone who may be in crisis. The emphasis, Lisa tells me, is not so much discussing their suicidal thoughts as being able to reach out to them – and say *anything*. The idea is that by simply commenting on the weather, you might be able to interrupt someone's train of thought and make them feel connected to somebody, which might be enough to delay a suicide attempt.

Chad's daughter Felicity says she has no doubt that her father would be immensely proud of where the organisation is today, especially the extent of their outreach services – to the homeless, prisons, schools and railways – and the use of technology like emails and SMS, so that listening is not simply done down the phone. But Chad's hope in founding the organisation has not been realised. He told the BBC in 1975 that he hoped suicide would eventually come to be seen as a 'highly unusual' cause of death – and yet it is still the leading cause of death for men aged between twenty and forty-nine.[57]

Samaritans has had a profound impact on my life. I remember in the early training, listening to a role play in which a man was weeping for his wife and family who had been burnt to death in a house fire. I was told, 'I can see you care, but I can't tell that from what you're saying.' I hope that over the past decade that has changed, and that I have become more adept at expressing compassion verbally. It has also given me a sense of the precariousness of life, and how quickly everything that seems solid can come crashing down. I have heard how easily things can change, and have been lucky enough to glimpse how transformative it can be if people are able to say things they had never imagined telling anyone. Perhaps, looking back, seeing how these stories could unfold helped me to tell my own story – to see, in the years to come, how it was possible to tell people things they were not expecting – and how to listen when they struggled to hear them. Perhaps.

But I am ashamed to say there came a time when I stopped volunteering. After nearly ten years on the phones, I realised I didn't feel the right compassion. I listened, but not as actively. The silences became lazy – a way of distancing and not reaching towards the caller. I felt anger when I saw the same people coming for face-to-face visits every other week. I could no longer listen to their stories openly and empathetically – and so I was not helping. In Eve's words, I was no longer 'useful'. So I took a break – for a while – but after a few months I realised I would not be going back. I am grateful beyond words that the service exists. But I felt as though I wasn't able to carry on; I was becoming robotic in my responses. I had heard too many stories – and the result was that I was no longer listening.*

---

* Samaritans are available 24 hours a day, 365 days a year. They can be contacted on the freephone number 113 126 (in both the UK and Republic of Ireland) or emailed at jo@samaritans.org in the UK or jo@samaritans.ie in the Republic of Ireland. For further information or to find your local branch see samaritans.org.

DANCING IN THE CONGO

FOR EVE, THE STORIES STOPPED in the Democratic Republic of the Congo, where she travelled in 2007 to see at first-hand the impact of the country's bloody civil war. The sheer scale of the trauma women had faced here floored her. More than half a million women and girls had been raped since the conflict began in 1996.[58] Rape had been used as a weapon of war to decimate villages, with young boys forced to watch as their mothers and sisters were violated. Here she encountered women – 'shaking women; weeping women; women with missing limbs and reproductive organs; women with machete lashes across their faces and arms and legs, women limping on crutches, women carrying babies the colour of their rapists, women who smelled like urine and faeces because they had fistulas – holes between their vaginas and bladders and rectums – and now they were leaking'.[59] For Eve, this conflict represented the endgame of neoliberal capitalism; the Congo was a place where mining the coltan for use in mobile phones collided with violence against women and the destruction of the planet.[60]

Back at her kitchen table, she tells me about the weeks she spent with a Congolese gynaecologist, Dr Mukwege, whose job it was to repair vaginas ripped apart in the course of a brutal war.[61] He would spend days working at the Panzi Hospital in Bukavu, sewing up women doubly incontinent as a result of multiple rapes. He agreed to let Eve speak to some of his patients. And she began to talk to the women who, despite these unspeakable traumas, were still able to 'dance when they could not walk'[62] and rebuild their lives in their tattered villages.

Inspired by these women, Eve helped to found City of Joy, an NGO and leadership school for women raped in the course of war, which every year trains women in how to reclaim their bodies and their lives and become leaders within their own communities: rebuilding the country from the inside out – and always starting with the women.

City of Joy opened in 2011, and its founding principles hark back to the essence of *The Vagina Monologues*, as the women learn how to look at their vaginas – squatting with mirrors and colouring pencils – to examine their bodies for the first time. Eve says that when the women leave they have a renewed sense of agency over their bodies. She remembers the first groups of women to 'graduate' from City of Joy.[63] They had decided their bodies were not for public consumption, not to be offered to men. For now at least. 'We said to them a few days before they left: "You are now healed, well, women and you have to be careful who you decide to give yourselves to, because you're golden." And they came back after a year and not one of them was with a man. And they said, "We haven't found anyone good enough." And at that point I thought, "We have been successful. We did our job."'

But the stories of generations of women have taken a toll on her. The words got into her bones and her body, and began to make her sick. In her memoir *In the Body of the World* she describes the destruction of Congo alongside her own diagnosis with uterine cancer. Perhaps it is a coincidence, but after decades of listening to the stories – giving people what she never received as a child – she developed Stage Four cancer that burnt up her uterus and vagina. It made her incontinent like the women she had spoken to in the Congo: connected up to stomas and bags. Her insides poured out of her; she developed a fistula. In a recent interview she said the women on the front line at the Panzi hospital had also got cancer[64] – these were the women listening to the stories of rape and death as the patients were checked in. It is a strange testament to the power of words.

Eve doesn't listen to stories any more. She has withdrawn to her house in the woods – or if not withdrawn, then at least she has redrawn the parameters of what she can and cannot withstand, the boundaries she lacked as a young woman, self-medicating with sex, drugs and war-zone adrenaline. She remains passionate about the power of storytelling – but listening to her speak you get the sense she now believes there is a limit to what one person can hear. 'I don't really listen to too many stories any more,' she says, 'because I did it for twenty years – and I'm very porous, and they just went into me. I cannot hear another story of violence.' She gestures towards her phone. 'My inbox, even now –' she struggles to find the words, 'oh my God, I get really really sick from it, I do, and I get raging, and I don't want to live in a state of rage.' She continues, 'I want the concrete now. I've been doing stories for twenty years.' She bangs the kitchen table. 'I want, "What are we doing?"' She pauses. 'We've got to go from telling to transformation. Telling your story will not solve all the problems; it will open doors, it will get things going, it will catalyse . . . but it's not the salvation.'

The salvation, for Eve, requires something else – before and above and beyond language. She glimpsed it in the Congo, while recovering from cancer, still sick and leaking from her own mended fistula. She remembers, 'I was really skinny and I looked really bad, I had no hair, and the women were so freaked out they thought I was dying and they all just started dancing.' But that dance was powerful. She laughs, 'I guess that's what everyone does when all else fails – and they were dancing so amazingly. I just thought, "These women have been through everything, and look how they're dancing. What if a billion women danced like that, what would happen, on the same day, what kind of energy would be catalysed?"'

This vision of women dancing for their lives became One Billion Rising – what Eve describes as the greatest mass action in human history. It was founded on the fifteenth anniversary of V-Day in February 2013. The idea is simple. According to the UN, one in three women will be subject to abuse in their lifetime – and at the time the statistic was calculated, that equated with roughly a billion women being raped or abused. Eve's idea was to get an equivalent number – one billion – to 'rise' to dance and reclaim public space to raise awareness of violence against women and girls and catalyse political change. The causes people 'rise' for are now more interconnected – for example, workers' rights and the environment – but, Eve says, these issues all coalesce in violence against women.

It is so easy to sneer at the idea that dancing could actually change anything in the world. But Eve says the impulse behind dancing is in many ways the same as speaking about the female body openly and without shame. Dancing allows women – or anyone – to inhabit their body. To claim it as their own. To move in ways that please them, without being cowed by work, or used for sex. If you know and inhabit and trust your body, then, the theory goes, you are less likely to let it be abused. As Eve explains, 'One Billion Rising is a way of people coming together in their bodies, because I think so much of what happens with violence against women happens on a landscape of our bodies, which is pre-verbal, which has no language – so we hold memories and self-hatred and shame and humiliation in our pores, and it really determines much of our existence. I think if you dance, collectively, something begins to happen where that starts to get released, and changed and redirected.'

She continues, 'For me it feels like that's when the revolution is going to happen – when women finally come back into their bodies. It is going to change how we see things, how we imagine what's possible. When you are separated from your body, you're separated from your motor, from the thing that's driving your life.' As a journalist, I am sceptical of these claims. I have built my life around the importance of speaking and telling, and it seems counter-intuitive that real healing would not be about language at all, but the pre-cognitive, primal movement of the body.

It is half-term when I arrive at a One Billion Rising event in Norwich. Crocuses are emerging from the grass verge beside the road and the city is busy with families. I wanted to see for myself whether dancing could really be as powerful as Eve had suggested, but there were no events scheduled in London, so I had to travel to East Anglia. When I arrive at the centre of town, a group of middle-aged women are beginning to set up the stage. They wear rainbow Dr. Martens boots and long woollen scarves over pink strappy tops. A few heart-shaped balloons are tied to a trestle table, and there are tubes of poster paint and plastic boxes of pens and glue sticks for people to make their own feminist placards. It has the air of a jumble sale. A small boy sits at the table eating Love Hearts.

Speakers take to the microphone to deliver polemics on domestic violence. They tell personal stories and quote dizzying statistics. But their proselytising leaves me cold. I know the violence is incomprehensible, but somehow talking about it is distancing. The woman behind the microphone feels different to me. Her story is not my own. People walk past, trying to avoid getting involved. During one of the particularly graphic speeches, a little girl turns to her father and asks 'What's that about, Daddy?' He is carrying a One Billion Rising sticker on the end of his finger – unsure where, or if, to stick it. 'I'll explain when you're older,' he replies as he guides her away from the crowd. And then the dancing starts. A younger woman leaps to the front and starts performing pre-choreographed moves, mirrored by about thirty others, in the manner of a slightly out-of-sync aerobics class. They are stamping and jumping in the cold. It looks fun. Silly. Shoppers stop to watch. A teenager leaps in, clowning and preening in front of his mates. A toddler waves her hands from her buggy, and two pensioners sidestep at the back of the group. There is something inclusive about the dancing. It invites people in, whereas the poetry and polemics push people away. I am beginning to understand. Removing language breaks down barriers – and perhaps having taken part in the dance you might be more willing to ask the organisers what the event is about. It is inclusive. That's why it works.

I wanted to meet Eve because I had huge respect for her storytelling – for the way she has broken down the taboos around the body by saying the unspeakable. But standing in Norwich, watching the dance, I am left with a sense of where stories fall short: the idea that, as Eve intuited, there is a point where words must stop or they can actually make you sick. I am drawn to this idea that there is something deeper than language, something in our pores which can't be expressed verbally. I want to know more about these stories – the ones lived in the body – and the places where words fail. But I am not a natural dancer, so I take pictures on my phone, and fade back into the crowd.

PART THREE

DEATH

KATHMANDU

THE FIRST NIGHT ALONE, I sleep wearing a whistle, the plastic ridge hard against my breastbone. Even five floors up, the night wheezes with the tireless swell of traffic. I have been filming in rural Nepal, and have decided to stay on by myself. I send the camera kit home with the rest of the crew – and now, for the first time since arriving in Nepal, I am scared. I wanted to stay on to try and find out more about how talking can help us process events. Since meeting Eve I have been thinking about whether speaking actually helps us to make sense of terrible things, or whether, as she intuited, there is a point at which all narratives run aground.

Lying in bed, I can't remember whether you should stay in one place or head outside during an earthquake, and in the dark I mentally trace the route to the street: across the stained wood floor and down the switchback stairs to the hotel garden. That would be the safest place. I have spent the afternoon speaking to survivors of the 2015 earthquake that killed at least 9,000 people here, and I now know that if, and when, it happens again, the death toll will probably be higher. The fact that the quake happened on a Saturday afternoon meant many people were outside, and the schools and offices were empty. One woman I spoke to told me how the water leapt out of the hotel swimming pool, sluicing frightened toddlers at a party. I press the whistle noiselessly to my lips, like a life-jacket demonstration before take-off. In a city of rolling blackouts – caused by electricity rationing or 'load shedding' – and a rat warren of narrow lanes, I don't fancy my chances.

Our driver had given the whistles to us two weeks earlier, outside Kathmandu airport. They are now standard issue for foreign journalists – handed out in the hope that someone will hear you if you were to be buried alive. Tired and disoriented, I pocketed mine, intent instead on counting the boxes of camera equipment from the porter's trolley to the car; checking the lights, tripod and lenses we would need for filming – relieved nothing had been lost in transit. An earthquake seemed a remote possibility, and I doubted how much difference a whistle would make.

But as we travelled through the country my views began to change. The signs of the quake were everywhere. On the drive from the airport, gaps like extracted teeth marked where buildings had once stood and mopeds picked their way between the poles that crisscrossed the street, propping up damaged façades. Piles of bricks were caged by chicken wire, ready for another day of reconstruction. Although the rubble had been cleared, rebuilding was slow, and in Kathmandu valley stairs reached Escher-like from ruined terraces, going nowhere, and families boiled lentils in corrugated iron shelters thrown up by international NGOs and never replaced.

The year is turning to the season of the quake again, and people are feeling jumpy. The weather is similar to April 2015 – colder than normal and unsettled, with sudden showers turning the dust roads to mud in minutes. Nepalese colleagues tell me they are attuned to the signs of disaster, and become startled by slamming doors or thunder. They watch the trees, in case the birds fly away in a sudden shudder, as they had in the moments before the tremor. I begin to ask people, almost vampirically, where they were during the earthquake and how they had survived in the months that followed. I want to understand what happened when the city was split open, and whether talking helped process the trauma of losing everything.

Some were almost untouched: one woman in her twenties was sitting in the cinema, and only found out what had happened when she turned on her phone in the foyer, to find dozens of panicky messages from her mother. Another, just a few miles away, was on her way home from the fields, and crouched in the middle of the road as her home collapsed beside her. She slept outside for days, too scared to approach the ruined buildings, before crawling through the rubble to retrieve her rice and pans. An American yoga teacher told me she made it to the doorway of her studio and stood counting the seconds of shaking – one, one thousand, two, one thousand – until she reached thirty, waiting for a thunderclap that never came. Aftershocks rocked the city for months, and I heard how people huddled in stairwells, or ended up spooning with strangers in overcrowded shelters, wearing motorbike helmets for protection from falling debris.

When the rest of the production team left, I moved across town to Thamel, the backpacker nexus of the city. Here, neon signs offered internet cafés and cheap international calls, the redundant precursors of the WhatsApp age. Tables laid with embroidered bags edged the streets, and cycle rickshaws replaced the shared taxis from the other side of town. Pollution has reached a record high, and everyone but the tourists wore disposable face masks. The streets should have been busy with trekkers stocking up on trail mix, but the stalls were quiet and designer knock-off anoraks turned slowly in the breeze. The risk of another quake continued to keep the crowds at bay.

But it isn't just the earthquake that has led me to Kathmandu. I have been here before. It is a place that changed everything for me – and finally brought me out of the isolation and celibacy of my twenties. A place where I began to reconnect with people. Lying in the dark, I remember arriving at this exact hotel, five years ago, long before the city was shaken. It still feels familiar. I delight in telling the waiters that I have stayed here before, and they show me around, pointing out renovations. The only obvious difference is that the communal computers have gone from the hallway and little stone elephants sit in their place on the desks where we used to email home.

I had come to Nepal to walk the Annapurna Circuit with my best friend, in the hope of crossing one of the highest trekking passes in the world. We arrived hot and jet-lagged, and spent our first afternoon sleeping fitfully in a pink room with orange curtains that diffused but did not stop the afternoon sun. Afterwards we sat in the hotel garden eating syrupy dal and discussing the days ahead.

At over 5,000 metres above sea level, the Thorong La is a remote belt of ice and rock strung high between the Himalayas, several hundred metres above Everest base camp. We had never climbed so far and were watchful for the symptoms of altitude sickness: the frothy pink sputum that would mean our lungs were filling with fluid, or the piercing headaches that preceded coma and death. While other trekkers compared photos in the evenings, we would rank our headaches from one to ten, and if they ever surpassed four, would split a chalky Diamox pill from the brown bottle we carried with us.

Our guide told us that a young Australian woman he had met at the start of his career had died from altitude sickness, and he wouldn't let the same thing happen again. He became the arbiter of our fate: deciding the span of a day's walking without a map and dictating when we should stop for the night. He laughed at our painfully slow pace, and would squat by the road to wait for us, trying to light a cigarette that never quite caught in the thin mountain air.

One of the chief symptoms of altitude sickness is hypoxia – a shortage of oxygen in the blood which can cause confusion. Often climbers won't realise that they are sick. The only way to prevent it is to stay where you are; halt the ascent, stop anything from changing. And despite our vigilance, a week after leaving Kathmandu, we fell ill. We were grounded in our guest house, and I sat and read while our guide joked about strapping my friend to a yak and carrying her down the mountain, 'Quick, quick!' The guest houses were transitory. No one but us stayed for more than a night, and the constant movement of people made time feel elastic.

Eventually we felt well enough to resume the climb. But my friend struggled under the weight of her backpack as she pulled herself along on the trekking poles from Kathmandu. I was furious; convinced that hypoxia was driving her towards death – and she couldn't see what was happening, although she had said she had a stomach bug. I railed against her decision to keep climbing, each step taking us further from the town – with its helipad and decompression chamber for climbers with the bends. When we reached the next tea house, she collapsed, tearful and angry.

But I had none of the open empathy I had proselytised about as a Samaritan. Something had shifted, for me, in the oxygen-empty air – and I had begun to see her differently. Perhaps the intensity of the fear and physical exertion had changed things for me. Or hypoxia meant I didn't know what was happening. I came to know the twist of her waist as we changed in freezing tea houses, and the slope of her back in the bed opposite. We never touched, but, to me, we were everything and nothing more than friends.

We christened our porter 'Paul Daniels', because of his penchant for magic tricks. Six foot tall in Green Flash trainers, he loped ahead. When we crossed the Thorong La, my friend hugged him. I stood in the snow as he threw his arms around her, holding her tired body tight. The last few metres had been tortuously slow, and I watched their embrace through the LCD screen of my new camera, forever stamped with the date of the crossing. Strings of prayer flags, brittle as moth wings, flapped in the background. I don't know why I didn't hug her initially – or why I didn't wait so that we could complete the crossing together. Perhaps I sensed there was something dangerous there – and had begun to pull away.

A year later we would kiss – almost twelve months to the day after crossing the Thorong La. And the flick of her tongue against my teeth confirmed something I had known for a long time. A physical, visceral truth – felt before it was spoken. Before I had come out and put everything into words. Before there was a story.

It was the first time I had kissed someone smaller than me.

We would continue to circle each other for months after that night, gnawing at each other's insecurities and nascent desire until I said something so unforgivable that she walked away into the night and didn't come back.

But this is where it began. In the dust of Kathmandu. I needed to come back here, to stand where we had been before it all changed; before everything was broken open and the world re-formed.

BUNGAMATI

THEY SERVE LUNCH EARLY IN Nepal. By mid-morning, Santi had already lit the stove and boiled the lentils for dal bhat. She was about to spoon the grainy mixture onto tin plates when the house began to move. Her first thought was for her husband. As is the custom in much of Nepal, they had been married when she was still a child and he was nearly twenty years her senior. A life of hard labour had turned him into an old man – the skin hung loose across his shoulders and his lungs gargled with TB. She didn't think he would make it out of the house in time.

We meet almost two years after the quake. It is only 11.30 a.m., but she is already clearing the lunch plates away. We are not the first people to come here asking for tales of the earthquake, and she doesn't offer us any food. My translator seems unsurprised. A young woman from Kathmandu, she has worked on countless earthquake stories and tells me how she sat in the doorframe of her apartment in downtown Kathmandu, filing stories on her laptop for international news agencies while others refused to go back inside. She has won a scholarship to study in the United States and won't be here long. Today she wears leggings and bright pink lipstick, with a gold stud in her nose, turning it whenever there is an awkward pause in the conversation.

Santi offers us small wicker stools and we sit outside, listening as she moves pots and plates just out of sight, behind a thin curtain. Their corrugated iron shed is at the edge of the main road and our stools balance on the banks of an open sewer. Recent rain has made the ground tacky, and the mud is papered with empty noodle packets, cigarette ends and a discarded child's sandal. After the quake, an NGO paid for Santi's youngest daughter to go to boarding school in Kathmandu, so she now lives alone with her husband.

He watches us, leaning on an upturned plastic water butt, as we wait for his wife. He is saying something unintelligible to my translator, who simply nods and smiles, as he fingers an empty blister pack of tablets. Flies settle on the untouched plate of dal beside him. I can't guess his age. Washing is hanging between the shelters, which back onto each other, with tiny gullies running between.

'They call these the cottages,' my translator tells me, looking up from her phone. 'Often earthquake survivors will still have their houses, but they're scared to go back inside.' She gestures across the road, to a row of red-brick buildings. Some are like dolls' houses, with the front blown off to reveal the outlines of rooms; signs of lives abandoned. Others are split by deep fissures floor to ceiling, or look half-finished, with the second storey missing, and stairs leading to the sky.

Santi emerges, wiping her hands against her cotton shift and apologising for the delay. She points up the road to where her house once stood. When it fell, they were too scared to go back inside, and slept in the open, until a local NGO offered them shelter. She never imagined they would be living in the hastily constructed 'cottage' for two years. The door is a piece of material strung between corrugated iron sheets – the cheapest and most readily available building material, which is burning hot in summer and mercilessly cold in winter. Bricks and logs are laid across the tin roof to stop it blowing away in the monsoon wind. Nothing tethers the cottages to the ground, instead they lean against each other on this small square of land.

Government grants have been slow to materialise here, my translator explains. 'There is no local government, so no one knew who to ask for help, or what they could get,' she says, touching her nose stud. 'So people are stuck.' The first of three tranches of government aid was paid to many families here earlier in the year, but Santi has not seen it yet.[1] She tells us that her rent keeps rising, so she can't stay here forever. 'She's right – this'll be valuable land,' my translator tells me, 'as it's so close to the city.' They are building a new road to Kathmandu, and behind the cottages a digger is working, watched by a crowd of children and teenage boys, as it carves a new edge to the village.

Bungamati is half an hour's drive from the capital, and barely distinguishable from the urban sprawl of the suburbs. Traditionally it has been an important ritual centre, home to a ceremonial chariot which is driven to the capital every year to guarantee good harvests and continued prosperity. In the months after the earthquake, the chariot was moved to and from Kathmandu as usual – but the town's main temple was destroyed and is now little more than a crater. 'They got the wrong bricks,' my translator tells me, smiling. 'Look,' she holds a brick aloft, to reveal the letters BVT stamped into the terracotta stone, 'these ones have lettering on them – so they're not right for temple-building. They're waiting for some plain ones.' She pauses. 'I guess it could be a long time.'

The demands of rebuilding are relentless, and Santi is busy. She takes our stools back into the cottage and asks if we would like to come and see her work. She hasn't the time to talk now. She pulls a piece of material from the clothesline to swaddle her face and mouth, and leads us through the gullies at the back of the cottages. Men sit in the sunshine, chiselling wooden window frames or carving the elephant-god Ganesh into soft lozenges of yellow sandal wood. 'The town is famous for its handicrafts,' my translator explains. And from the cottages we can hear the rhythmic thud of metal hammers against tightly woven wool, as women weave carpets to be sold to the tourists in Thamel.

'It's good they had their handicrafts,' my translator says, 'at least they had a way to make money.'

The town still attracts tourists. A ghoulish procession is making its way along the main road, and we can see their guide's umbrella held aloft as we cut through the terraces. 'Looks like they're still growing crops,' my translator gestures, indicating rows of improbably green wheat and what look like spring onions.

After a few minutes Santi stops. We are standing in front of what was once an enormous house – two storeys, with a balcony and iron metalwork on the windows: evidence of money and the years spent building a life. This is where she will work today. She leaves us standing outside listening to the crash and fall of construction. When she returns, she is carrying plastic chairs and cups of sweet black tea. We are told to sit and watch.

Brick by brick they are dismantling the houses, finishing what the earthquake could not do. The bricks are needed for new buildings, and those left half standing are unsafe for human habitation, so their owners must tear them down. Today Santi will carry bricks from this house to another pile a few hundred metres away. She will earn a handful of rupees for her labour. I am struck by the paradox of dismantling lives when there is still so much rebuilding to do. There is no wrecking ball of corporate construction here; it is the women who do these jobs, often pulling down the houses, without the capital to rebuild. The men work in Kathmandu or, like her husband, are old and infirm. She is Sisyphus, physically shouldering the impossible labour.

It's a pattern repeated across the country, I'm told. A few days after meeting Santi, I speak to the head of Nepal's Transcultural Psychosocial Organisation, which promotes mental health here. He tells me not just the physical but often the mental and emotional burden falls to women. With their husbands away, they must do everything: raising and rebuilding families and homes destroyed by the quake – and yet they have almost no role in the decision-making process, thanks to the enduring patriarchy. It is funny how once again my research has led me back to the women – and that it is women who do both the physical and emotional labour of rebuilding. 'It's an imbalance,' he says, that can make life 'intolerable'. I am shocked to discover that suicide is now the leading cause of death in women of child-bearing age in Nepal.[2] But when I tell people here about this statistic, no one else seems surprised; it is simply an indicator of how tough life can be.

My translator and I sit in silence, drinking the sweet tea and watching Santi slowly moving the bricks across the damaged land. She is joined by three other women, who move quickly and mechanically, with their wheelbarrows. No one speaks as they work because of the dust. I hold my phone up sheepishly to take a picture. Suddenly my reasons for being here feel absurd. I am a shameful voyeur. How can I ask her how she has processed the trauma of losing everything when the loss is still so new and the imperative is to rebuild, not to ruminate? Nevertheless, I have come this far – and feel I need to try – to understand how people here have processed trauma and whether talking is helpful.

I nudge my translator, who calls her over. 'Didi,' she shouts above the noise of construction. The phrase, meaning 'sister' in Nepali, is used to refer to any older woman. Santi sets down her load and walks over, unwinding the material from her face. My enquiries feel hopelessly crass. I hear the words in my head before I say them: 'Could you tell me what it was like when the earthquake hit?' She looks confused, and I am glad I can hide behind the translation. I stare at the ground during the bubbling

Nepali that follows. Santi's feet are brick-dust orange in plastic sandals. Squinting against the sun I flinch at her answer.

'She says it was very hard,' my translator says. There is a pause. The translator looks up enquiringly, touching the stud in her nose. 'Is there anything else?'

I reel off the symptoms of trauma I have read about, hoping to prompt a more effusive answer: 'Was she able to sleep? Or – easily startled?' I grasp at examples: 'Were there memories of the event that threw her back into the moment of impact – so it felt like it was still happening?' My translator nods and turns to Santi, and the stream of Nepali resumes.

'She says they couldn't sleep.' She shrugs, 'But that was because everyone had to sleep outside, as there were so many aftershocks. And yes', she continues, 'she says she was scared. Is there something more?' my translator asks again, squinting against the sun.

I am deflated. 'No, that's fine,' I say. The gaps here are too great. I'm not sure if it's the phrasing of my questions, the quality of the translation, or the absurdity of asking any of this that shuts the conversation down. I press my hands together as a mark of respect and finish my tea.

In the taxi back, I wonder how I am going to do this. Of course there is no time for talking, or to analyse your coping mechanisms, when you are pulling your neighbour's house apart brick by brick so you can afford to pay the rent on borrowed land. There is no time to talk through how things have affected you, or recognise the symptoms of trauma, when you are scrambling to survive and you still can't trust the ground beneath your feet.

I turn to watch Santi through the back window of the taxi, as she tips the bricks out of her barrow. These are the lucky ones – with a stream of reliable income and close to the wealth of Kathmandu. But still they have no time to talk.

SHELL SHOCK

THE IDEA THAT YOU CAN talk your way out of trauma is relatively new – and perhaps I am naive in thinking that it would be even remotely applicable to the situation in Nepal. I remember reading how, in the aftermath of the Rwandan genocide, well-meaning psychologists arrived to try and heal the psychological scars of war, and were sent away. According to the writer Andrew Solomon, the idea of sitting alone in a darkened room during therapy was incomprehensible to the Rwandans: to recover you needed to be outside in bright sunshine and with the community. The idea of being separated from others and forced to talk about what had happened to you, alone in a dingy little room, was believed to be profoundly damaging.[3] And yet the power of the talking cure has shaped how we, in the UK at least, view traumatic events and how best to recover from them.

I first learnt about the development of the talking cure at a Samaritans annual conference. A military historian showed us grainy slides of the victims of shell shock – and explained that the respect with which we now treat many aspects of psychology emerged from the experience of war.[4] He showed us slides of men who had come back from the front during the First World War, and were unable to return to battle. Their symptoms were diverse, but were collectively known as 'shell shock'. Often these symptoms would affect their speech: some were stuck dumb, others were unable to remember where they were or what had happened.

One of the photos showed a man twisted in a wheelchair – with no apparent physical injury – his body simply unable to cope with the horrors of war. He was called Percy Meek, a basket-weaver from Norfolk who was invalided out of the army with shell shock two years after signing up.[5] He had had to be restrained from running towards the German front lines, and when he reached the first aid post he was unable to speak and was hallucinating that he was still in the trenches. When he arrived at Netley hospital in Southampton he was still unable to talk and could not stand without support.

Men like Percy posed a problem for the authorities as they were bed-blockers who cost money. The British establishment had to find a way to get them to process these unspeakable experiences, so that they could return to battle. In the end it was 'electric shock' that restored Percy's speech, but physicians also tried hypnotism and occupational therapy to restore his words – as well as the talking cure.

The phrase 'the talking cure' was first coined by Sigmund Freud's colleague Dr Josef Breuer and was used to describe the treatment he performed on Bertha Pappenheim, or as she was known in the case histories, 'Anna O'.[6] In *Studies in Hysteria*, Freud explained that talking therapy could help to cure a patient of their hysterical symptoms, by allowing them to access a deeply buried hurt, something so traumatic that the brain had submerged it in the subconscious, only for it to surface via inexplicable physical symptoms. Freud wrote: 'We found, at first to our great surprise, that the individual hysterical symptoms disappeared immediately and did not recur if we succeeded in wakening the memory of the precipitating event with complete clarity, arousing with it the accompanying affect, and if the patient then depicted the event in the greatest possible detail and put words to the affect.'[7]

These theories came to be of crucial interest to British military personnel trying to solve the enigma of shell shock – and get men like Percy Meek back into active service. One proponent of this new method was the psychologist C. S. Myers, who wrote the first paper on shell shock,[8] and maintained, as Freud had suggested, that the brain split off from things it couldn't deal with and that the men needed to regain 'volitional control' of the repressed events 'if [they were] to be healed'.[9]

George Oppen's war experience also had a profound and lasting effect upon him. Even decades after the recognition of shell shock as a medical condition, he still seemed no better equipped to process what he had seen. He fought for the Allies during the Second World War in France and was injured in the closing months of the conflict. Linda, his daughter, remembers how, in the years after Oppen's return from the war, her father would often need to feel that there was a wall behind him and that Mary would go into crowded rooms ahead of her husband, to clear a space for him. It was a time of unspoken psychological damage: 'The silence was my only memory of his returning home,' she says.[10] As a child, Linda also remembers how the house had to be kept dark and quiet when Oppen came back from France, and that she would often find him wandering the house after a nightmare. It seems he kept revisiting the battle-fields by night long after he left the front lines, for Oppen wrote that he had two definitive dreams in his life: the first was of rust in copper, and the second was that 'I shouldn't be trying to kill people'.[11]

Oppen circles the war experience again and again in his poetry, seemingly tormented by what he saw – but never, explicitly, telling us what happened:

> in the destroyed (and guilty) Theatre
> of the War   I'd cried
> and remembered
> boyhood   degradation   other
> degradations and this crime I will not recover
> from that landscape it will be in my mind[12]

I learn what happened to Oppen during those final months of the conflict from the words of one of his friends. In an essay written after Oppen's death, David McAleavey explains the cataclysmic event which haunted Oppen for years afterwards, for he says that Oppen found himself trapped in a foxhole under direct fire.[13] The men he was with had already been injured, and lay bleeding beside him. Oppen realised that one of the men could only be saved by being carried across the open fields to the first aid post – which would have been suicide during the attack. So he chose to save his own life. He pulled the man's injured body over him, for protection – but not before the man had realised Oppen had chosen not to save him or drag him to safety. Perhaps this is part of the guilt that seems to plague Oppen, and which surfaces again and again in the poems: he knowingly did not save someone – not only that, but he used their still living body as a human shield. It must have been an impossible situation for this ethical poet who thought long and hard about his actions.

In his poetry Oppen goes back to the foxhole time and again. There is something important in the experience, and in the retelling of it – working through the why and how:

> Wars that are just? A simpler question: In the event,
> Will you or will you not want to kill a German . . .
>   Why
> Did I play all that, what was I doing there?[14]

This guilt at why he went, leaving his young family, was to torment Oppen throughout his life – as he writes in the daybooks:

> My disguised volunteering into
> the war: it was absurd. It
> Was perhaps a time in which what
> One did could be absurd. Or worse
> Than absurd.[15]

But while he talks at length in his poetry about the decision to go to war, and his guilt at fighting, he circles, but never takes us directly back into the foxhole. The events there are left for others to tell. Perhaps it could never be purged through poetry. Reading Oppen's war writing I begin to wonder how you could ever recover from these experiences – and if talking, writing, reconfiguring and painstakingly refracting it into literature is helpful.

In the case of shell shock it has been well documented that talking did, undeniably, make a difference, and the war experiences led to profound change in the way psychiatry was practised in UK.[16] Hysterical symptoms were no longer seen as simply a female affliction; and there was finally a significant financial investment in investigating the links between mind and body. The First World War eventually led to the opening of several specialist psychiatric hospitals – and in some sense paved the way for the enduring idea, enshrined by Samaritans, that it's 'good to talk'.[17]

HEALING THE HEART-MIND

I AM EMBARRASSED BY MY inability to talk to Santi, and I retreat to a Western-style café in Patan, the smarter end of the city. I understand the signs and symbols here: wifi, gluten-free brownies and banana lassis, and I know my language will work. I can get what I want – the communication is simple and transactional.

Something about my isolation reminds me of the Oppens in Mexico. They didn't learn Spanish and barely ate the food. They were neither one thing nor the other, cut off and at one remove from the local people.

I have come to the café to meet American anthropologist Liana Chase, who is studying how people are engaging with mental health services introduced in the wake of the disaster. She has just been trekking in Sindhupalchowk, one of the most severely damaged districts, and is wind-burnt and tired when we meet. A snowstorm left her stranded in the mountains for days, sharing a local teahouse for shelter. She sits, curled in a black hoody, and orders her coffee in fluent Nepali, her earrings jangling as she speaks.[18]

She tells me the scenes in Bungamati continue up the mountain. 'There is a lot of suffering,' she says, 'but not necessarily trauma; it's more social issues triggered by their living conditions – and by not having any money.' Alcoholism has increased, and the anxiety of trying to rebuild has taken its toll – family relations can be strained, and the incidence of abuse has risen, as it always does when times are hard. It's well documented that during economic downturns the levels of domestic abuse increase – with women once again bearing the brunt of change.

She tells me Santi's stoicism is typical, as there is a widespread acceptance that suffering is just part of life here. 'I think part of it is that in these Buddhist communities, there is a belief in the idea of *dukkha*.' She explains to me that *dukkha* is the first Noble Truth of Buddhism, that life is inherently unsatisfactory, and that therefore suffering is unavoidable. This *dukkha* can only be overcome by enlightenment, which releases you from the cycles of earthly existence.[19] 'What's important,' she continues, 'is that this means suffering, loss and grief are all normalised – not pathologised.'

In her experience, this normalisation of loss and struggle means that people are willing to talk about their experiences openly. 'There's this whole body of work,' she says, 'about how Nepali people are not able to talk about emotions – but I don't really buy into that.' The problem, she says, is that Westerners use the wrong language to begin the discussion. I think of my own fragmented conversation with Santi and cringe.

Central to getting people to 'open up', she explains, is understanding that feelings of distress are not talked about in the same way as they would be in the West. Crucially, in a Nepali setting, the idea of 'mental health' doesn't make much sense, as according to the Nepalese notion of self, feelings of distress do not originate in the brain, as neuroscience teaches us, but in an organ called the 'heart-mind', or *man* in Nepali.[20] There's nothing quite like the 'heart-mind' in Western physiology, but it sits in your chest and is where emotions and some forms of thought are experienced. In contrast, the 'brain-mind', or *dimaag*, in your head, is where logical thought and decision-making take place.[21] Disorders of the 'brain-mind' are deeply stigmatised in Nepal. Whereas tension, or *tanaab*, in the 'heart-mind' is understood to be part of normal life. There is a risk, Liana says, that if you try to talk about trauma using Western idioms, you will not only scare earthquake victims, but unintentionally isolate and stigmatise them. It would, in short, be the worst possible way of trying to start a conversation. My questions to Santi now feel desperately naive: I was using the wrong language, the wrong idioms, and even the wrong concept of suffering and what it is to be a person.

The conversation is further complicated, Liana tells me, by the fact that suffering is often somatised in Nepal – or experienced in the body, rather than through the emotions. So instead of talking about feelings of distress, people will complain of stomach aches or fatigue. 'A lot of it revolves around physical symptoms,' she says. 'People will say, "My wife feels dizzy" or "She forgets things". Lots of people talk about numbness and tingling – they call it *jhum jhum* – in the fingers and legs. There's quite a consistent list of symptoms that people talk about that may not map onto PTSD as we would understand it.'

What's exciting for Liana – and what has drawn her to Nepal for her research – is that these Nepali ideas about self and suffering have led to a new form of grassroots, culturally adapted, mental health support that doesn't exist anywhere else in the world. Following the end of the ten-year civil war here in 2006, she tells me, there were 'all these local NGOs popping up', tasked with helping former child-soldiers and civilians recover from the conflict.[22] Using local idioms like tension in the 'heart-mind', alongside an understanding of somatisation, they developed a form of counselling that is tailored to the Nepali context and which continues to be widely used. There are subtle differences from Western models of talking therapy, so that in Nepal you would not make eye contact, or sit directly opposite a client during counselling, and 'they might also spend three days talking about *tanaab* or tension, rather than depression'.

The result of this was that when the earthquake hit, there was no flood of well-meaning foreigners offering psychological support, as they had done after the tsunami in Thailand or Sri Lanka. Instead, local people were able to provide locally adapted talking therapy. 'The old narrative of Westerners going in and kind of imposing their models doesn't really hold any more,' Liana tells me. Instead, there is a 'new era of post-disaster mental health intervention'.

This 'new era' goes beyond straightforward talking therapy to something called 'psychosocial counselling', which sees mental health as the product of environmental factors. According to Liana, people here are not interested in simply talking about their problems – and any discussion must sit alongside alleviating the physical causes of distress, be they poverty, alcoholism or abuse. 'There is a problem-oriented approach to dealing with mental health issues here,' she says. 'If you know someone is stressed because of a family situation or an economic situation then you need to look directly at addressing the source of the problem, rather than just talking about it.' Part of this is recognising that psychological distress isn't simply an unspeakable internal affliction, but is the nexus of everything that is going on: emotionally, socially, economically – and no one is depressed in a vacuum.

This model of psychosocial counselling has been pioneered by Nepal's Transcultural Psychosocial Organisation (TPO) – founded just as the civil war was ending, and now dedicated to improving mental health across the country. Liana tells me there is nothing quite like it anywhere else, and that they have developed networks of local women who will go house to house in the villages, offering 'psychosocial support'. In practice these women offer something akin to Samaritans' active listening, and are trained 'not to go too deep', but to listen and then refer any difficult cases to local psychologists, who can in turn send patients for more specialised care.[23]

A few days later I meet the head of TPO Nepal, Suraj Koirala, and he echoes what Liana has told me about the importance of not mentioning mental health here. 'When you talk about mental health, you know,' he begins, 'they will imagine a person without clothes, a person with a lot of aggression, a person locked in a room or held with a chain, and they will not think mental health applies to them. We approach it in terms of symptoms – because anyone can have symptoms, like you can't sleep, or you don't want to talk with others. That's something that people can understand. We say this is a "psychosocial issue", not a "mental health issue".'

He tells me that after the earthquake his teams discovered much lower levels of PTSD than they had expected.[24] But, unlike Liana, he doesn't put this down to religion – but to politics. 'In my opinion, people here were resilient because they are not expecting anything from the government. If people had nothing before, then they don't expect anything afterwards. They don't wait for handouts to start rebuilding.' I suspect he may be right. It is well documented that having a sense of agency can help to limit your experience of trauma – and one of the things that tends to lock people in a cycle of depression is a feeling of being powerless and trapped.

The challenge, Suraj explains, is convincing policymakers that talking therapy is worth the investment. 'When you go to a district, and are coordinating with the different agencies, you have to put in a lot of effort to make people understand the importance of psychosocial counselling. People are much more likely to want to spend money on houses or new bridges.'

But, he says, there is hope. Despite the devastation, Suraj believes the earthquake could still change how people think about mental health in the long term. The disaster brought renewed funding and a greater interest in counselling and psychosocial support. So more people are starting to talk about their problems.

I return to my hotel to go through my notes as the city shifts into the early evening. Women on adjacent rooftops collect their washing and stop to check their reflections in mirrors stuck to open walls. A man carries an Alsatian down a fire escape from its pen on the roof, and a young boy practises archery – shooting fibreglass arrows into a fixed target, inches from pots of geraniums. I feel very alone.

The idea of feeling trapped and without agency reminds me of Oppen – perhaps what saved him both psychologically and physically was pulling the body on top of him, so that he was physically able to do something and claw back a modicum of control.

And I am beginning to understand how misguided my attempts to talk about the earthquake with Santi were. This is a culture of deep resilience, where years of political instability and civil unrest have taught people to fend for themselves – and where deep-held religious beliefs dictate that suffering is inevitable. And, when people are willing to talk about their feelings, they bear no relation to the Western model of distress. The things I had imagined to be solid, like selfhood and suffering, are not fixed – and without the local language I have little hope of getting to the heart of how people have coped with the trauma of losing everything. As I'm beginning to realise, it's not simply a question of not speaking Nepali – it's not understanding the things that make you human here.

Perhaps the best way for me to understand how people artic-ulated their distress would be to talk instead to the people who *listened* – the volunteers and psychiatrists who helped in the weeks after the quake, and who understood what to ask and how to let people tell their stories. I increasingly feel that my westernness, and credentials as a British journalist, get me access and then promptly get in the way. I need to move myself one step further from what was spoken, to try and get closer to what was said.

FLOWER AND FLINT

I AM STANDING OUTSIDE THE main hospital in Patan. It is rush hour, and commuters skid past on motorbikes, anonymous in visors and face masks.

I've come to meet Damber Lata, or 'Lata', a young woman who was involved in a pioneering study into the power of story-telling after the earthquake. I am worried about meeting her after the disappointments of Bungamati. Our initial communi-cation has been confused – half-formed text messages tapped out on an old Nokia – and I'm not sure what to expect. A woman pulls up in front of me on a motorbike and flips her visor away from her face.

'Harriet?'

She hadn't mentioned the motorbike. It seems I am incapable of asking the right questions here. She pats the leather seat behind her, without removing her helmet, so we can go some-where and talk. I climb on reluctantly, and as we dive into the Kathmandu traffic I feel painfully British, holding her anorak gingerly between forefingers and thumbs, as I don't want to hug her middle for stability. I close my mouth against the dust. Lives bleed into each other here – street vendors' shops open out on the road: blacksmiths, fruit stalls and newsagents selling melted chocolate and nappies, stacked against the counter. We are miles away from the capsule living of London, where cars and shops are discrete entities.

I remember learning how some South Asian cultures are thought to be collective, so that personal identity is bound up in your relation to others, and you are always someone's daughter, mother or sister before you are yourself. Here, as we jump over the speed bumps and pull alongside whole families on motorbikes, it feels as though we are part of the city itself. It reminds me of Foucault's Panopticon – the prison where everyone behaves because they are being watched by everybody else; each a part of the others' lives.

We arrive at a brightly painted children's home in the suburbs, where Lata now works.

We sit in the administrative office, at the top of the building, looking out across the rooftops of Kathmandu. After the earthquake, Lata tells me, she desperately wanted to help. She slept in a hastily constructed plastic and bamboo shelter for a few days before leaving the city to stay with relatives, and when she came back life had almost returned to normal. She resumed her Masters in Psychology, and was enjoying studying, when her course leader asked if she would be interested in joining a clinical trial, looking at whether talking therapy was an effective way of processing trauma.

It was the first time Lata had ever put any of the theory from her research into practice, and as she sat down in the garden of the hotel she was nervous.[25] Her first client was a woman in her early twenties, who at first seemed desperately shy. She wouldn't meet Lata's gaze, and stared resolutely at the floor. Lata wasn't sure what to do, so she poured her a glass of water and waited.

Lata was part of a pioneering study into Narrative Exposure Therapy (NET), a form of talking therapy in which a patient tells their story in minute detail to try and restore equilibrium to their memory of events. Research in the wake of other natural disasters had found it was cost-effective and seemed to help the victims to recover from trauma. So in 2016 a group of Nepalese psychiatrists and psychologists, from both Kathmandu and the UK, developed a clinical trial to test its efficacy in Nepal.[26]

Suraj Shakya, a softly spoken man, was Lata's supervisor and responsible for recruiting volunteers for the trial. One Saturday morning he explains to me how talking in explicit detail about traumatic experiences can help speed recovery. He first used NET with a young woman who had been abused and was struggling to cope – she was suffering overwhelming flashbacks. 'I told her I wanted to hear what had happened to her as a story,' he says. 'I asked her to try and pinpoint exactly what she was doing, and how she felt at each moment.' When Suraj had heard her story, he wrote down every detail and then read it back to her. Her experience had been transformed into a neat artefact: words on the page, contained and controlled. 'Repeating the story, the pain becomes less – it becomes less hot,' Suraj tells me. 'She has pain still, but it's not that big hot memory. The main thing is to expose her to the story again and again so those hot memories become integrated.'

It is well documented that trauma affects our ability to tell stories, to create a narrative with a fixed beginning, middle and end. Trauma messes with time, so that events from the past intrude into the present in violent flashbacks, nightmares and panic attacks. Brain scans of trauma victims during flashbacks show that they are not remembering an event from the past, but are reliving it.[27] Suraj tells me that the aim of repeatedly retelling the story of traumatic events during NET is to try and ground the events in the past. He gives an example from his own life – in the months following the earthquake, he would panic if he heard dogs barking, and would start sweating and feel his heart racing as if he was living through an aftershock. At first he could not understand it, but after going over the events of the earthquake in painstaking detail, he realised that just before the first tremor, the dogs in the neighbourhood began to bark. Once he had realised that this sound was triggering his panic, he was able to make sense of how he felt and, over time, his fear decreased.

The process of NET starts with a lifeline – giving the chaos form by laying a ribbon on the ground, so the story has a definite beginning, middle and end. When Lata was faced with her first client, they sat in silence for most of their early sessions. Then Lata laid a ribbon across the table in front of them. She placed a small plastic flower at one end of the ribbon. 'There,' she said, 'that is where you were born.' The woman was intrigued. Lata showed her a box of plastic flowers, and urged her to take more. 'These are the good things,' she said, 'and this ribbon is your lifeline. You can put these flowers on the lifeline, whenever a good thing happened.' The biggest bloom was laid towards the end of the ribbon. She told Lata it represented the birth of her daughter, three years ago. Lata then asked her to gather a handful of stones from the garden. These were different sizes, from shards of gravel to rocks big as a fist. These stones were to represent the more difficult events of her life.

To Lata's surprise she placed a small stone on top of a flower. 'That is my marriage,' she said. She had been married young – a love marriage, unusual in her village, where most nuptials were arranged by the couple's parents. But she had chosen a lower caste boy. And when she married, her family disowned her for her unsuitable choice. She moved in with her in-laws, as was the tradition. But this was the beginning of her troubles.

It transpired it was not the earthquake itself, but the chain of events that followed, which had made life unbearable. When the earthquake came, the family survived, but their house was shaken to the ground, and her in-laws blamed her when no one came to help them rebuild. She was meant to have brought wealth and prosperity to the family – but their fortune lay in ruins. Ignored and shamed by both her own family and her in-laws, she began to feel desperate. Her husband stopped speaking to her, and her mother-in-law was increasingly cruel – physically and emotionally beating her. There was barely enough money to survive. She began to cry uncontrollably and lost interest in the rituals of family life.

One day a group of women came to the door with a survey,

asking people how they were coping. They had a checklist that tallied with her life, and the cycles of sadness and desperation. They explained that they were providing free counselling in a local hotel – would she come? The young woman slipped out after making the family meal one morning. She didn't tell anyone where she was going. She didn't know how to explain that she was going to talk about her sadness with strangers.

She plucked a rock from the garden and laid it on the ribbon. It was larger than the others, rucking the fabric. Ah, thought Lata, this will be the earthquake – the source of hot memories which refuse to stay in the past but break through to the present, so that as soon as you mention them you start to relive them, shivering and shaking as though the roof has fallen in. But it wasn't the earthquake. The greatest sadness in her life had occurred long before. Her sister had been trafficked to India – sold by a relative to help support the family. This was the greatest rock on the ribbon. The unspeakable thing. Decades of sex-selective abortion in India mean there is now a shortage of girls, and people-trafficking to meet the supply – for brides, prostitutes and domestic servants – is surprisingly common.[28]

She had never told anyone about her sister, and she sobbed as she told Lata about the way she had disappeared. There is no doubt in Lata's mind that having the opportunity to speak was a good thing. There had never been anyone in the girl's life who had been willing to listen before, and somehow the experience of being heard, and seen, as a person – and not simply a means to an end: a dowry, a mother, a maid – was important.

As Lata speaks, I am reminded of a widow I once filmed in Afghanistan. There, widows are seen as the lowest of the low – morally corrupt and untouchable – 'a pot without a lid', to coin the local idiom. She was in her sixties, and her husband had been killed by the Taliban, decades earlier. Since then she had earned a living sluicing the blood from a hospital floor; she raised her children alone, as she was never allowed to remarry. Her son was about to join the Afghan army, as there were no other jobs available, and she was braced to lose him too. At the end of the interview, she thanked us. 'No one has ever asked me how I feel before,' she said, 'about this pain in my heart.' It was such an unremarkable story of poverty and war that its humanity had been overlooked. It was only recovered in the little details: not saying goodbye to her husband the day he died, and the fact his grave had been washed away in a flood. Several commissioning editors turned the film down before they saw the finished tape, saying 'We've heard it all before'. But no one had heard her story before, and there was a value in the telling. I understand why Lata feels there is something powerful about listening to these women – the lives lived just below the surface, which were cracked wide open by the earthquake, so they couldn't ignore the injustice and isolation any more.

I ask if, after only two days' training, Lata was worried about re-traumatising the girl. But she shakes her head. The change in her was remarkable, she tells me. After four sessions, she was able to make eye contact and speak without crying. She hadn't been to school and couldn't read or write, so Lata wrote her life story down and gave it to her to keep. It was a physical emblem of the work they had done. She said she would keep it and then give it to her daughter, who was going to go to school. She would be able to read it. She would have a future.

But despite Lata's optimism, the clinical trial was never completed. The team simply couldn't get enough data. Suraj Shakya, who ran the trial together with professionals from the UK, shakes his head when I ask him about it a few days later. 'There are so many things we could not have anticipated,' he sighs. Suraj doesn't know if it was the act of storytelling that put people off or other external factors. 'We were only a small team,' he says, 'we didn't have enough people, and we were only volunteers.' Resources limited the team to Kathmandu valley, rather than allowing them to travel into the mountains where the need was more acute. And even in the relative security of the suburban towns, the team weren't able to tempt enough people to come to the local hotel, where they were based, to tell their stories. Perhaps the journey to the hotel itself was the problem. He mentions elderly women, who would need to be chaperoned at the therapy sessions. His team couldn't provide the extra bodies – and the ever-pressing needs of subsistence farming meant it wasn't practical to come back time and time again to talk through events of the past.

In some ways it was heartening to hear the basic truth I discovered at Bungamati held here too – that survival takes priority over storytelling. The UK leader of the trial, Dr Arun Jha, is even more dismissive when I speak to him over the phone: 'These people, they just suffer!' he says. But he also concedes that this suffering may not be alleviated by talking to a strange man in an unknown hotel on the outskirts of town. 'They rely on traditional healers – the shamans, the witch doctors, to help them,' he says, 'and they have their families. There are very strong communal ties, so if someone is withdrawn, or suffering, it will be noticed much earlier than it would be in the UK.'

Perhaps it was just circumstance that meant the trial failed. It was too far to travel to the therapy sessions, there were too few trained therapists, too few hours to return time and again to tell the same story. And yet, as I listen to Suraj, I begin to wonder if there is something about storytelling itself that puts people off. If there is in fact something about these experiences that disrupts our ability to keep the past behind us, that resists stories. Perhaps there are things for which we just can't find the words.

NOBODY WOULD EVER PRINT IT

I UNDERSTAND THE IMPULSE TO tell stories, the need to narrate an event so many times it stops being real. As soon as my friend and I kissed I began constructing a story, scaffolding the raw feelings in facts and explanations, to try and give my emotions form. Stacks of old diaries bear witness to the telling.

A phrase from Roald Dahl rumbled around in my head as I wrote, 'I dare not write it, even hint it, nobody would ever print it!' The 'it' refers to the expletive Goldilocks utters in *Revolting Rhymes* when she breaks Baby Bear's chair by 'plonk[ing] her fat behind' down too fast. This was the terrible, unspeakable truth: I liked women.

I worked through all the people in my life, trying to explain how I felt. I couldn't say the words yet: gay, lesbian, dyke – and bisexuality sounded like a medical condition. So I mumbled the stock phrase 'I like women' over and over.

The first person I told was my mother. I remember turning my mobile on to speakerphone and putting it on the windowsill, the morning after the kiss.

'Hi, it's me,' I said. My voice sounded very small.

A framed photo of my four siblings sat on the otherwise empty bookcase opposite. In it we were sitting by the Christmas tree, in matching jumpers. I must have been about eleven and was holding my baby brother. Soft-faced and wide-eyed, he was laughing. Our hair lit white-blonde by the flash.

'I'm sorry,' I began, 'I'm so sorry. I need to come home.' I clenched my jaw to stop myself from crying.

'Oh darling, what on earth has happened?'

I slid down to the floor and sat wedged between the bed and the bookcase. I was grateful that the phone was on loudspeaker, and I didn't have to hold it against my face. There was something reassuring about being contained in the small space.

I told her my friend and I had kissed, running the sentences together, so there was no room for query or question. 'We have been so close that it's turned into a pseudo-relationship.' I said. 'And I want it to end.'

'OK.'

I could have stopped there. But I knew if I didn't tell her then, I would never find the words.

'I think I've been unfair. Maybe I've led her on. Because I think I like women. No – I don't think it, I know it. I like women.'

My mother's voice was high and tight when she answered. 'I've been preparing myself for this. After you came back from Nepal, I started to wonder, and . . . well, I'm not surprised.'

And somehow her words took the revelation away from me – diffused it and dampened it, by telling me she already knew.

'I feel like I've let you down,' I said. 'I know this isn't what you want to tell your friends.'

'No. But we'll get used to it.'

But I didn't want her to get used to it; to be accommodated and tolerated. I wanted her to acknowledge the enormity of this revelation, and how much it scared me.

I moved home for a few days after that call. Before I unpacked, I went into my grandmother's study, seizing control of events, so that my mother would not be the one to tell her.

'I wasn't expecting to see you here, dear,' my grandmother said as I came in, and patted the sofa.

'Yes, well, it's been a bit of a mad week,' I replied. 'I think that my friend's in love with me.' We looked at each other.

'You're right – that does sound a bit mad,' she said. 'And did you know she was that way inclined?'

'No. The thing is, though,' I paused, 'I think I might be that way inclined.'

'Right. Well. There you go.' She leant forward and closed the *Radio Times*. 'I suppose it's better that you can be honest about it. Just look at Clare Balding,' she said, gesturing towards the muted TV, 'she seems so, you know, normal.'

She hurried on. 'Of course I've known lots of people like that – my first husband's butler was a queer. He made me give him the sack because he said it was an abomination, and the poor man just cried and cried.'

The following weekend we were sitting outside together in the afternoon sun. My sister's guinea pigs were in a mesh cage on the lawn, and the dog prowled around them, worrying the wire with her teeth.

'She'll go for the jugular,' my grandmother said. 'They're trained killers, terriers.'

My father was clearing the gutters as we ate, his hands full of blackened leaves. The coleslaw had begun to sweat in the heat and I got up to take it indoors.

As I turned, my grandmother looked up from the *Sunday Telegraph*. 'I don't think you should wear that skirt any more Harriet,' she said. 'It makes you look very butch.'

Later she cornered my brother and told him how she had watched a lesbian sex show in Paris in the 1940s. She told him about dildos and fucking and how repulsive she found it. Then she asked my mother, as they were driving to Tesco, if she was really going to let me back in the house. My brother relayed these conversations to me weeks later.

'You should never have told her,' he said. 'No one wants to have a conversation with their eighty-seven-year-old grandmother about dildos.'

Each new disclosure became part of the story – a tissue of reactions and exclamations. I would explain about travelling in Nepal and the shift I felt in the mountain air – and then give the quick reveal that 'I like women too'. A confusing and comedic twist. My grandmother's comment about dildos was relayed with a smirk to old schoolfriends, and I told earnest colleagues of the early conversation with my mother.

In the months after coming out, I looked back through the photos of the trip, trying to make sense of what had happened.

My album was full of bright images of blue skies and prayer flags. I stopped at a picture of two chortens, the hollow stone monuments erected at the holiest points along the trail. Neither of us were in vision. None of the pictures told the story I remembered, the elusive truth of what actually happened.

And so I continued to tell and re-tell until I could gain ownership of events. But each narration drove me further from myself. Everyone laughed at my grandmother's reaction – but all I felt was sad, grieving the loss of my imagined future. My story was hollow: a paper rose, folded into itself with nothing in the middle. My feelings weren't there – it was just a list of things that happened. Frost-bitten fingers and the date stamp on a camera screen. I never found the words to say, 'I am lonely.'

As I listen to Lata and Suraj explain Narrative Exposure Therapy, I can understand how re-telling would cool the hot memories, and re-integrate them. I think in those early days I was trying to build a new self, making sense of how I felt through a narrative – the only way I knew how to construct meaning. But it didn't work. In those lonely hours I needed to be touched, to be held. Not to tell stories.

'TRAUMA DOESN'T LIVE IN THE story.' Yogatara leans forward, conspiratorially. Her arms are slim and crossed, her short blonde hair falling into her eyes. We are sitting in The Summit, one of the smartest hotels in Kathmandu. Everything is dark wood and marble. It is nice to be among the diplomats, rather than the backpackers of Thamel.

I've come here to meet Renee, a Dutch psychotherapist who has lived in the city for nearly a decade, and has helped both Westerners and Nepalis deal with the fallout of the quake. When she arrives, she is leaning heavily on a crutch following a recent car crash, and has brought a friend, Yogatara, a fellow Kathmandu ex-pat, for support. As soon as we begin talking about the quake, Yogatara becomes animated, leaning forward in her seat and pushing her sunglasses onto her head.

'The story is not enough,' she says, 'there's a place for that, but it's not enough. Trauma lives in the body – and until it can be resolved, in the body, it will never go away.'[29] She is incredulous about the idea of using Narrative Exposure Therapy in a city still rocked by aftershocks, where people are in the midst of the process of rebuilding. 'With trauma, when you tell the story you physically re-live it,' she says, 'so it could trigger all these responses, and you could easily be re-traumatised.'

Even two years on, it is clear that neither she nor Renee feel completely secure here. Renee is in the process of moving back to Holland. There are other issues, she tells me, problems with work visas, the education system and pollution – and the continued threat of another quake looms large.

She leans forward. 'I don't want to say it too loudly,' she says, 'I don't want to scare people, but we live on a fault. It will happen again.' She glances around the bar. 'I was in Rotterdam last year to have my second son, and I was at the top of this big building, and every half an hour I would panic, and then realise I was safe again. You shouldn't need to realise you're safe. You should know it. It's just a given.'

'Do you remember where you were when it happened?' I ask – the question somehow seeming less clumsy with fellow foreigners.

'I was here!' Renee replies. 'I was sitting over there, at the bar, and I'd just ordered my apple pie from that guy – I call him my earthquake waiter.' It was King's Day, she remembers, so everyone was wearing orange. 'It's a strange Dutch thing!' she laughs. The children were running around the pool with their faces painted, and the adults were hazy from an afternoon of slow drinking. Renee was looking after her son, who was still a toddler, 'So I wasn't drinking actually,' she clarifies with a smile. Suddenly she had a strange feeling. 'It was as if I was really hungover, even though I hadn't been drinking. I looked at my friend across the bar and she had this terrible expression, and I just knew.' She pauses, gesturing at her route to safety. 'I stood up, and I thought maybe people will think I'm stupid, but I'm doing it anyway, so I grabbed my son and shouted "Earthquake!" And when I got to the doorway the shaking started.' She looks outside to the terracotta patio, where waiters are carrying coffee. 'I just remember putting the pacifier in my son's mouth as we fell to the ground.'

'When did you feel safe?' Yogatara asks, presciently. I am speechless.

'When I saw my husband in the car park,' she says. 'People were still panicking, though.' The water from the swimming pool was rising up in claps, splashing down over the families, fuelling their fear.

'It really changed everything for me,' Yogatara agrees. She now looks for escape routes as soon as she enters a room, and has dedicated herself to helping other survivors. 'Helping others has been a big part of my own recovery,' she says. But it is a slow process. She admits she is still jumpy, and that months after the quake, a banging door could send her straight back to the moment of impact. Her normal coping strategies, like yoga, didn't help initially. 'People talk a lot about feeling "grounded" in yoga, and I was like, fuck you, I don't trust the ground!'

Her outlook changed when she met an American trauma specialist, who introduced her to the idea that some traumatic events could be processed without recourse to traditional talking therapy. Lisa LaDue was a Red Cross veteran of 9/11, the

Thailand tsunami and countless fires and hurricanes – and used a method known as somatic experiencing. The name comes from *soma*, the Ancient Greek for 'body'. I think of Suraj and his patients with physical symptoms. So much here seems to come back to the body.

Somatic experiencing, or SE, is, Yogatara explains, based on the way in which animals respond to traumatic situations. It was developed by psychologist Peter Levine, who noticed that prey spend their lives fleeing capture, but remain calm and relaxed when not in the heat of the chase. They are not plagued by traumatic memories of these near-death experiences in the way that human beings so often are. He speculated that we could learn a lot in our treatment of trauma from the animal kingdom. His breakthrough came in 1969 when treating a graduate student called Nancy, who suffered paralysing panic attacks. One day, during therapy, Levine suddenly had the image of a tiger crouching to stalk its prey and urged Nancy to 'See the tiger as it comes towards you! Run! Climb up! Escape!' Nancy immediately and involuntarily began to pedal her legs, as though she was physically running away, before shaking uncontrollably as she 'escaped'. This visualisation of the escape from the tiger was the beginning of Nancy's recovery – and of Levine's development of somatic experiencing.[30]

'It's like an antelope,' Yogatara tells me. 'When they're being chased, they either get away, or they don't. If they know they're not going to get away, then they freeze – and then there are all these chemicals in the bloodstream to numb them. If the threat leaves, then they'll come out of that freeze and they'll shake

– just shake the adrenaline and cortisol through their system and then run off. But we get stuck. Instead of shaking, we'll go "Oh, I shouldn't cry, I shouldn't yell. What will everyone think?" Our "thinking" brain gets the better of us. That's how we end up traumatised.'

She is speaking from painful experience. In the months after the earthquake she couldn't shake herself to safety, but was in a state of continual anxiety. 'It was the aftershocks,' she says, 'you never knew when they would come, or when they would end.' She spent the first few days camping in her garden, digging a trench around the tent to keep the rainwater out and texting her father, who was a former US Marine, for moral support. 'I kept waiting for someone to rescue me,' she says. 'As a child I was taught the Marines would come and save you, so I was subconsciously thinking, "The Marines are coming, the Marines are coming."' She pauses. 'But I was alone.' It was only when she began learning about somatic experiencing that she was able to breathe again.

I am ashamed to say that talking to Westerners has made it real – and I sleep with a whistle that night. Like Yogatara, I mentally plan my escape – how I would leave the hotel if the worst were to happen. Death seems closer than before I met them. One of Yogatara's parting thoughts keeps running around my head. 'The hardest part,' she said, 'was to know that so many people had died in the same place at the same time. It felt as if they had lost their physical bodies and didn't even know they were dead yet. The energy was like a wave – this energy of death.'

The next day I walk down to Pashupatinath Temple where the city's dead are cremated. In the months that followed the quake, Pashupatinath became an emblem for the unthinkable loss of life. The fires by the river burned continuously as the victims were cremated. Thousands of bodies were burnt on the ghats by the Bagmati river. The ghats are five minutes from the international terminal at Tribhuvan Airport – so death is always in plain sight. Perhaps part of the reason people coped so well in the weeks after the quake was that death is such a visible part of life here. The bodies are burnt in public, and this life is, according to both Hindu and Buddhist traditions, just one of many. The end is nothing to be feared.

When I visit, the water is little more than an inch high. Children wade across, picking at the dregs of plastic bags that float on the surface with sticks. A body draped in red lies by the river. I read in my guidebook that cremation should happen as soon as possible after passing – so these are the newly dead. Families arrive carrying polythene bags of fruit and flowers. Four ghats are smouldering, and men poke at the ashes with poles. Another is newly laid with criss-crossing slabs of white wood. The ground is blackened by the flames. A few tourists watch, circled by guides and mangy monkeys, all hoping for something. Cremation at this holy Hindu site is meant to expedite the journey of the soul to the next world. Watching the saddhus sitting by the smouldering pyres, I am reminded of Yogatara lying in her tent, listening to the chanting coming from the monasteries across Kathmandu valley to speed the passing of the deceased. Mourning the dead is a slow process, marked by ritual and music. In the Buddhist tradition it takes several days for the soul to pass into the next realm, and the monks chant to ease the dead from the earth, as a strange peace descends on the broken city. The physical moment of death is in many ways immaterial.

I've only recently started to understand that death is a process, rather than the final full stop, beyond which nothing can be said. My first real experience of loss was the death of my grandmother.

At the end, the barrier between life and death was gossamer thin; and her last breath seemed an arbitrary marker. She died a week before Christmas, following a massive stroke. But there were ciphers that outlived her: her handwriting remained on the blackboard in the kitchen – 'Oil for the counters; washing up liquid'. I don't know who wiped the words away eventually, or moved her glasses from the kitchen counter and closed the medical dictionary left open in her study. I assume it was my mother – who tried to close her eyes after she died – but couldn't force them shut. The day after her death I was standing with my mother in my grandmother's bedroom, when the lights flicked on. No one was near the switch. In the weeks that followed, my parents had to get a new kettle as it kept switching on spontaneously and the lights in the house would fuse in the middle of the night. I understood Yogatara's feeling for the energy of death.

When my grandmother died, I knew from the start that I wanted to see her body. We had to leave the hospital almost immediately after she passed – to make room for the next person in an overstretched geriatric ward. I remember the smell of her day-old hairspray and the touch of her rapidly cooling skin as I kissed her goodbye. My grown-up siblings had all come home during the day, and we had sat in her hospital room, taking turns to get coffee or sandwiches. Whenever my mother left the room I was terrified my grandmother would die, and I wouldn't know what to do. I sat watching her rattling breath, feeling utterly ill-equipped to deal with death. In the end, the movement from life to death was almost imperceptible, eased by the morphine, and my mother, who told her not to be scared. That we would all be fine. That she was loved – and there was nothing more she needed to do. She opened the window so her soul could fly out. We drove home squeezed into the people carrier, just like when we were small – my brothers' knees almost against their chins. The sky was lit bright pink by the setting sun, and we all looked out of the car windows at the fading light and the dark branches against the horizon. No one said anything; we just watched the farewell swoop of colour move across the sky. When we got home I made spaghetti bolognese for everyone. We opened a bottle of wine. It seemed unreal that she was gone. I wanted to see her – to be sure.

The laying out was in a chapel of rest behind the undertaker's, in a car park just off the high street. The undertaker led us in. There was a small holding area before the room where the body had been prepared.

'She's just in there,' he said, his hand on the door handle. 'Are you ready?'

She looked at once herself – and totally different. My mother and I had chosen what she should wear: the flattering pink jacket and matching skirt. The undertaker didn't ask us to provide shoes. I didn't like to think why. I walked to the edge of the coffin and felt the firm cold of her thigh under the woollen skirt. Her skin was so smooth. In death, the wrinkles of her face had relaxed. She would have liked that. But some of the colours were wrong; her fingernails had become dark lozenges where the blood had stopped. And as I stood there, I remembered hearing how the undertaker glues a corpse's eyes and mouth together for the laying out. When I told my sister she left the room crying. I'm not sure why I said anything. I think I wanted to fill the silence.

My grandmother died before I could tell her that I had got engaged. My parents had admired my new ring as we stood by her hospital bed. I wanted her to know. In the years after my coming out, she had simultaneously developed a soft spot for my girlfriend while maintaining a horror of our sexual intimacy. 'I'm engaged,' I whisper into the room. 'We're going to get married.' It was strange to be met with silence. It reminded me of the poem from so many years ago – about speaking to the silent dead. The poem that I had read out in the Speech and Drama competition. The poem that had helped me to find my voice. Speaking to the dead is perhaps the safest – and most futile – form of communication. No one is going to say anything back. There will be no congratulations, no raised eyebrows, no judgements passed after the event. I simply wished she had known.

I didn't know what else to say. So I recited a poem, whispering it into the silence. It seemed fitting. I was due to read the poem at her funeral the following day. She had chosen it herself, in the years before her death. She had had plenty of time to plan what should be said to mark her passing, and had picked poems for each of us to read. She had always been so proud of us, even when we were children. It was important to be able to read it without crying: I didn't want to make a scene. I read it again and again the week of her death, until the words didn't mean anything. 'Because I have loved life,' I began, whispering into the silence, watching her expressionless face, 'I shall have no sorrow to die. / I have sent up my gladness on wings, to be lost in the blue of the sky.'

When I had finished, I walked out of the chapel of rest into the car park. My siblings had gone around the corner to have coffee. I stood and looked at the sky. It was the most beautiful bright blue day.

Another line from the same poem haunts me in Kathmandu, as I am speaking to the earthquake survivors about death. It is the final thought, in which the speaker concludes, 'I know that no flower nor flint was in vain on the path I trod.' It is on my tongue as Lata tells me about the plastic marigolds and pebbles placed on a length of ribbon to mark the span of a life. And for a second I am choked. Through these strange coincidences I have thought about my grandmother almost every day since she died. I hadn't realised until now that the relationship would carry on, in spite of her death.

As I watch the families at Pashupatinath speeding their relatives to the next world, I realise that the next person I speak to must be someone who can bridge that gap over the great unspeakable and talk with the dead. It is time to see a shaman.

The first problem, though, is that no one wants to help me find one. Many of the people I have spoken to have told me that shamans, or witch doctors, played an important part in helping people to recover from the quake. But no one could point me in the right direction. They are elusive – universally alluded to, but just out of sight. I ask my translator over the phone if she knows of anyone. 'No,' she says, 'I've asked and no one knows.' I'm not sure if she is being elusive because she is embarrassed by the presence of this traditional hocus-pocus in her modern city. In desperation, we return to Bungamati to ask Santi if she knows of anyone I could speak to. I follow my translator between the tin cottages, past a scarecrow with a bin-bag body drooping down to the ground. Santi is working at the same building site, still moving bricks from place to place, and we speak against the continual sound of breaking rocks.

'Didi,' my translator begins, before disappearing into a stream of incomprehensible Nepali. Santi listens and nods. She pulls the material from her face and gestures across to the other side of town, to the largest building still standing. My translator turns to me with an incredulous smile. 'That's so lucky,' she says, 'she says she does know someone. She never went to see anyone for herself, but she went for her husband – to see if they could help with his TB. Shall we go?'

The house Santi gestured to is three storeys tall and stands beside a near-stagnant pond. Ducks with mangy patches of naked skin paddle at the water's edge, picking their way through the mud-caked rice packets and cardboard. My translator leads the way, asking at each floor if they know where we can find the shaman. Different families live on each level, and we step over men sitting cross-legged in the hallway, chiselling at unfinished window frames. The smell of the fragrant wood chips rises above the standing water below. I'm not sure what to expect when we reach the top floor. A woman in a red cardigan and what was once a matching red wraparound skirt is leaning against the balcony, watching our ascent. Her cardigan is a few sizes too small, and her body strains against the buttons. She has tucked her phone into the waistband of her skirt, and runs her fingers along the edge as we approach.

'This is her,' my translator says. 'They call her the god of smallpox – as she has the gift of healing.'

I press my hands together in greeting and, after a few words of Nepali, she leads us into an adjacent room. It is a shrine room of sorts, and she gestures for us to sit on the floor, in the far corner, away from the ceremonial objects. Laminated posters of Hindu gods are pinned to the oppressively pink walls, above a makeshift throne, and the floor is scattered with grains of rice. Drums are stacked in a dusty glass cabinet beside the throne, and a collection of gold lamps, urns and model hands reaching skyward in supplication are arranged around the shrine. I ask if it might be possible for her to demonstrate how these objects are used, but the goddess shakes her head – Sunday is her day off.

I realise that she is first woman I have seen here who is

inactive – not cooking, washing or carrying. We sit on the floor, legs tucked beneath us, as she explains her craft. Through the translator she tells me that when all the other buildings fell in Bungamati, her shrine room survived. She was sitting on her throne at the moment of impact, and had to be carried out through a window. She is now in her forties, and says she has never received any formal training in her craft – but equally has never had any complaints. She doesn't pretend to understand medicine, and says that for many people that come to her, all she can do is send them to hospital. Rather than a doctor, she seems to be the village confessor. Women come to her, she says, looking for reassurance. They often come if their husbands are drinking heavily and they don't know how to make them stop. In these cases, she says she will make offerings for them, or will offer to perform a *puja*, a form of religious ritual. She is affronted when I mention the comparative luxury of her multi-storey house, and ask if she is paid for her services. She tells me she is never given more than a few rupees at a time – or perhaps an offering of beans and eggs.

Around the time of the earthquake she was busy. People would come with physical symptoms, like headaches or indigestion – the somatic aches and tics that belie a trauma so deep it can't be expressed. She tells me many people came to her because they were being haunted by relatives who did not survive the quake. The answer to everything seems to be offerings and *puja*. She doesn't ask to hear anyone's story – but in exceptional cases, where people are particularly distressed, she will ask them to sit before her and sprinkles them with rice and holy water – the trappings of baptism and marriage – to herald a new world, free from pain.

As we leave, I still want to know more about how these shamanic rituals work. The Bungamati shaman seems to offer little more than a kind word and reassurance, but I've heard that shamans are often called on to heal deep trauma – the kind that can't be cured with words and a handful of rice: a sadness so severe it is as though part of your soul is missing; it is known colloquially as 'soul loss'. I can't see that the self-styled mother goddess would be able to deal with this level of trauma, and so, a few days later, I am in another taxi, winding my way through the suburbs of Kathmandu.

In the end I gave up on authenticity and settled for a feted shamanic school, where Westerners are taught these ancient traditions. At least, I reasoned, the teachers there would be used to explaining their practices to foreigners. On the drive to the centre, the dust collects around my mouth. The taxi driver is agitated, shouting at the proprietor over the phone and muddling the directions, so that we end up outside a school playground, watched by inquisitive children. Eventually a man in a tweed flat cap and matching jacket comes to find us, and we follow his moped to the iron gates of the shamanic centre.

Subin Rai now runs the centre, and leads me through the garden to a monumental dark stone grave.

'This was my papa,' he says, gesturing towards the picture on the headstone. 'He set up this place.'

'I'm so sorry,' I say, as he leads me towards the house.

'Why?' he replies. 'Death is part of life. He has gone, but he is with us.'

Subin comes from a long line of shamans. His grandfather was a shaman in the royal court of Bhutan, and passed his craft down through the generations. But, he tells me, there are other ways to learn this form of dark magic. An elderly woman with a lazy eye brings us cups of weak tea, and sits down beside us for a cigarette.

'That's my auntie,' he says. 'She's a shaman too. But she wasn't taught by our family – she was taken by the Banjhankri when she was nine, and he taught her. She has been a shaman since she was thirteen.' The old woman nods, although Subin tells me she doesn't understand English. The Banjhankri, Subin tells me, are wild shamans who traditionally live in the forest, and abduct children to teach them the art of shamanism. According to shaman mythology, they are terrifying creatures, part man part bear, with backward pointing feet and long matted hair like a monkey. His auntie smiles, and wanders off towards the open kitchen door, where a small child is pottering in a baby-walker, and a man with dreads washes pots in the sunshine.

Subin tells me that shamans believe that man is part of nature, and as such should protect the environment – almost like God's steward in Eden. According to this worldview, bad things happen as a result of simple natural law: if you poison the air, then the fruit will rot. Subin is emphatic that nature is a benevolent force, and mankind needs to live in harmony with his environment – but we can't quite get to the bottom of what he believes caused the earthquake, or how the movement of tectonic plates fits into his theology.

He tells me he was leading a group of German tourists on a pilgrimage to a shamanic shrine when it happened. They saw houses 'break apart and come together, break apart and come together', as the land shook. In the hours that followed, the group pooled their medical kits to provide crude first aid to the villagers. Initially there was nothing he could offer, as a shaman, to alleviate the physical suffering, but once he was back in Kathmandu, he began to treat people for 'soul loss'.

The soul is divided into several parts, Subin explains, and if you are particularly afraid a piece of your soul can break away. This would usually happen while you are sleeping, as the soul travels at night, and if your sleep is disturbed, then part of your soul could get lost and be unable to find its way back into your body. If part of the soul is lost, he tells me, then people become tired, irritable, unable to concentrate and no longer seem like themselves – displaying all the hallmarks of what we would call depression. It is the shaman's job to tempt the soul back into the body. As he speaks, I am reminded of Suraj's efforts to reintegrate experience and put his clients back together through storytelling. Everyone is trying to mend what has been broken apart. But Subin's healing is not about words so much as physical contact and sound: the beat of a drum and skin on skin.

'Could you show me how you do it?' I ask.

He laughs. 'How? We do not know when people will come needing soul-retrieval. We must wait for them to come to us.

And we do not know when the powerful shamans will come here from the mountains. You must wait.'

I think of the taxi-meter, turning over outside the gates. I don't have time to wait. And besides, two years on from the quake, the people seeking help are few and far between.

'Maybe we can do some ritual with you?' he suggests, sensing my agitation. 'We can see how things are with your health – and with the ancestors – something like that?' Clearly he is used to dealing with inquisitive, and monied, foreigners, and once we have exchanged a handful of dollars, he leads me towards the house.

My insides clench as he leads me inside. We have agreed on a small ritual to give me a sense of how a shaman would perform a healing. He leads me into the main shrine room and asks me to sit on the floor. It is welcomingly cool and dark here. One wall is covered with images of gods. Some I recognise: a seated Buddha, leaning to touch the ground beneath him, a crucifix and a marigold-garlanded Ganesh. Others are unknown: wooden masks, painted red with curling mouths, a knitted witch strung from the ceiling, and dark glaring gods bearing swords. The floor is laid with ceremonial objects: a dish with burning incense, hollow tortoise shells and a human skull.

His auntie will perform the ritual. She begins by holding one of my arms, and then the other, above my head, pressing her thumbs deep into the soft tissue at my wrists, as if searching for a pulse. When she has finished, she mutters something to Subin.

'That's very good,' Subin says. 'Your health is fine. But she says there is a problem with your father's ancestors.'

'OK.' I am still sitting on the floor, looking up at him like a supplicant child.

'She will do a ritual now, to help the ancestors,' he says. And with that, he leaves us.

The floor is cold under my crossed legs, and instinctively I keep my gaze lowered, watching the aunt's feet as she prepares the ritual objects. She has left her sandals by the door and is wearing socks embroidered with tiny bows. She hands me an engraved wooden dagger with a grunt, pressing it into my breast-bone and closing my fingers around the hilt, to show me how to keep it still. She collects what looks like a twist of rope, a few centimetres long, and holds it against a burning nub of incense. The rope crackles and begins to smoulder. She lifts it out of my view and stands directly in front of me, as she begins to chant.

The music is low and stumbling. I can't make out any words or tune as such – it is more a guttural, pulsating thrum. I can almost feel the heat coming from her body as she stands before me, waving the twist of rope-like incense in and out of my view, spirals of smoke twisting skywards. My senses are height-ened by the almost-touch, just as when someone brushes past you on the bus, you never quite know when the next contact will come. She touches the incense to my forehead, smearing the ash with a thumb. I am attuned to the heat, the movement and sound from another body. Then she starts shaking. Her heavy wooden beads and bangles clatter together, and the humming rocks in her throat. Her hand is warm on my shoulder as she presses into the muscle, and shakes me, gently and rhythmically, for a few seconds. She ends the ceremony by pressing a small gold jug on my head. The ring of cold metal is heavy and soothing. Without a word she walks from the room. The sounds of metal being scraped and the smell of boiled rice drift into the shrine room through the open door. It is lunchtime.

I know the ritual is superficial; $20 and a few minutes with some frightening effigies – probably nothing more than a show for the tourists. But there is something very good about being touched, after days alone in the city, asking endless questions and being asked nothing back. It feels good to have something to hold onto, and to feel my skin prickle with the heat of incense and shiver of metal. It is the first time anyone has touched anything other than my right hand in a week. I can feel the blood tingling in my fingers as I set the dagger down and involuntarily roll my shoulders, pressing my thumbs into my shoulder blades, where I was held.

Subin escorts me from the centre, with instructions to remember the dead. His aunt is smoking, and waves as I climb into the taxi and trundle back towards town.

I can still smell incense in my hair, and wipe the ash from my forehead in the rearview mirror. I hate to admit it, but there was power in that dark room. I may not have been suffering soul-loss, but already my body feels more attuned to physical sensation: the hot naked metal of the car door and the bone-jumping bumps in the road. The physical act of being shaken surprised me. It reminds me of Yogatara's description of the antelope, and the idea that movement can help to shake the fear from a terrorised body. I think perhaps she is right, and that there is something about touch which could help to alleviate the isolation, and fear, of deep trauma – if this glancing contact with a stranger has already made me feel more alive.

THE SHAKES

'WE WERE DRIVING TOWARDS THE bullseye,' Lisa LaDue smiles. 'I mean, the Pentagon was literally just there – like a target.' She leans back and laughs. Something about being in danger seems to trigger her laughter, and I wonder if perhaps her humour is what has enabled her to survive the litany of trauma she has witnessed, first as a Red Cross volunteer, then psychotherapist, and lately through her work with somatic experiencing. She shows me bright holiday snaps from her disaster work. There she is after the tsunami in Thailand, beaming, with her arm around an indigenous woman on a beach. Here, with Hurricane Katrina survivors, squinting at the camera.

'I learnt pretty early on that I thrive in emergency situations,' she tells me. 'I was working in the Emergency department, and I suddenly thought, "Oh no – am I one of *those* people?"' She laughs again, 'Am I some kind of adrenaline *junkie*?' she pauses, serious suddenly. 'But you know, you don't work there to feel like that – you work there because you *can*. Not everyone can do it.'

I meet Lisa just before leaving Nepal, and we talk in Yogatara's kitchen. She is only here for a few months to visit Yogatara, and hopes to continue her work with earthquake survivors – although bad weather in the mountains has so far made it impossible to reach the affected communities.[31] The sun is blistered through the mosquito mesh at the windows as we talk, and my feet are cold on the marble floor. Lisa is a wonderful storyteller, smaller than me, and perched on her chair like a bird.

She tells me her life changed after the attack on the Twin Towers. In the days and weeks after 9/11 she was asked to help support the Red Cross effort, and was drafted in to help with the disaster response. She was not speaking directly to the bereaved, but even away from the front line, death was inescapable. 'You would walk out of the elevator, and there would be someone saying they'd just gone to identify their son,' she says. Part of her role was to help educate people about the effects of trauma. 'I was saying to the firemen,' she pauses, 'because I'm a volunteer firefighter myself – you need to watch yourself. You could be digging up body parts at Ground Zero during the week, and then your wife will say "Oh honey, could you help me in the garden?" And that could be enough to trigger you.' It was, she says, a strange, twilight existence, working all hours and then falling into bed. 'We were being driven to the Pentagon by a different route each day, with armed guards,' she says, 'so there really was an elevated sense of *risk*.' She had worked as a 'first responder' with the Red Cross in hurricanes in Puerto Rico and Guam, and thought she knew about trauma. But this was different.

During the day she functioned normally, providing high-level briefings and peer support. She noticed that when she got home in the evenings, she might feel a little depressed, but she assumed it was just the adrenaline draining away. But once the work at the Pentagon had finished, she started to notice that although she wasn't consciously thinking about 9/11, her body was still processing what had happened. 'I found I couldn't sleep,' she says. 'I had no difficulty falling asleep, but I would wake up at four in the morning.' She wasn't master of her own body any more. She remembers one day, a few months after the attack, she was at a presentation when an image of the Pentagon flashed up on a slide. 'I just started crying,' she says, 'tears were just running down my cheeks. I couldn't stop.' She later developed tunnel vision and found she couldn't see colleagues even if they were in the same room.

'I had a few long dark nights of the soul,' she says, 'and I realised I wasn't in a good place.' But what scared her more than the sleeplessness and tunnel vision was that she didn't know how to help herself. 'My training is in cognitive behavioural therapy, or CBT,' she explains, 'so we're taught that the way to change your behaviour is to challenge the way you *think*. According to CBT, if you can change the pattern of thought, then you can change the way you behave. But this time it didn't work.' She pauses, cradling her coffee in both hands. 'This was somewhere deeper. I wasn't looking at the picture of the Pentagon and *thinking* anything – the tears just came.' Lisa was scared. 'I thought that was it,' she says, 'I thought my career was over, because not only could I not help myself get better

– I realised that what I had been doing may not have helped anyone else either. And no one I knew could help me, because everyone saw trauma the way I did.'

Faced with the prospect of losing her cherished career, Lisa began to research trauma, and her reading soon led her to Peter Levine. 'I went to a traumatic studies conference,' she says, 'and I heard him talk about how he had helped a woman who had been buried in the rubble – and what he said resonated with me. It made so much sense to me that trauma lives in the body – not in the mind.' She began learning how to practise Peter Levine's therapeutic method, somatic experiencing, and found that her symptoms began to subside.

'So how does SE work?' I ask. And here we run into trouble – as every attempt to explain the technique, which is grounded in the body, rather than in narrative, fails.

'Maybe it's easier if I show you,' she says.

'Now, try and remember something mildly traumatic,' she suggests, and promptly laughs. 'Nothing too drastic – how about being stuck in traffic on the way here?' I smile, remembering the dust and tinny taxi radio. 'Right, now I want you to notice how you feel in your body, right now, as you think about being stuck in traffic.'

There is a small stirring in my gut and I uncross my legs. 'There,' she says, triumphantly pointing at my feet on the floor, 'you may not have even noticed it, but by having both feet on the ground, your body is better placed to get away. How do you feel now?' I shrug. The shifts have been so subtle I felt almost nothing. Lisa nods, and suggests that during this small demonstration I should have experienced how it feels to be agitated, and then almost immediately have become aware of the reassuring cool marble underfoot as my body responded to feeling threatened. This is, she says, similar to somatic experiencing, when a client is encouraged to notice how their body feels during a traumatic memory, and then is trained to notice how it feels to be in the present moment – creating the realisation that they are safe, so their body can relax. There is something powerful and reassuring about the physical sensation of being safe, she says, which can break the cycle of trauma.

But creating the sense of safety can be almost impossible after an earthquake, when the ground beneath your feet is not to be trusted. 'I never use the word grounding,' Lisa says. 'Instead, I use the word "anchoring", and it might not be about feeling your feet on the floor – I might ask them to hold onto the back of the chair. It just has to be something solid. Being held can help too,' she continues, 'whether it's your arms or someone else's, it doesn't matter – your brain can't tell the difference – it just responds to touch. A warm blanket is the most useful emergency response tool. It's not about thinking, "Oh this reminds me of my mother", it's more basic than that, it just builds a felt and experiential sense of safety.' Trauma, Lisa tells me, doesn't live in our cognitive, storytelling brain. In fact, brain scans of trauma survivors during flashbacks show that the language centre of the brain physically shuts down during these terrifying events.[32] Instead, trauma lives in the older, more primal region of the brain which governs the fight-or-flight response before we have time to think. If the body feels safe, she says, then the feedback loop will tell the reptilian brain there is no danger and the flood of fear will ease.

The beauty of this technique, Lisa explains, is that there is no need to re-tell the story of the traumatic event; rather, the body is encouraged to realise the threat is in the past, so that it can relax and start to heal. It works in an international disaster setting, she says, because there is little need for language, and the to and fro of translation. Almost a year after the earthquake, she tried out somatic experiencing techniques in one of the most severely affected areas. There she met a man she calls 'the headmaster', whose son had been buried alive in the rubble. As a community leader, he was responsible for helping to organise the reconstruction work, and for supporting others. But he wasn't functioning. 'He had this glassy stare,' Lisa says, 'it's something you see a lot in trauma. People get stuck in freeze mode – because that's how they survived, especially if they were trapped some-where. They'll often tell you they don't feel happy or sad, and they're just emotionally flat, until something re-triggers them, and then they're out of control and might have flashbacks or panic attacks.' She shows me a picture of the headmaster jumping over a skipping rope. 'Look at him, stiff as a board,' she says. His hands are balled into fists, and his hat is still on his head as he leaps into the air. Looking at the photo, I wonder how appropriate it is to ask a traumatised community leader to start skipping in front of his peers – and whether Lisa would have done the same if he was an American politician. Perhaps she would, for as she explains, she knows that sometimes she has to overstep cultural boundaries.

'When he came to see me,' she says, 'I asked if I could hold his feet, which I know isn't something a Nepali woman would do – but he said OK,' as her foreignness seemed to allow her to sidestep the rules. She explains that many people who are traumatised will have little awareness of physical sensation in their bodies, and so touch can be a powerful tool. 'Sure enough, he couldn't even feel his feet,' she says, 'they were physically numb.' As she held them, the feeling gradually came back into his toes and he began to move away. 'I said, "Stay with me." I could see he was uncomfortable, but then he laughed, and there was a physical connection between us.' The feeling of discomfort had actually helped to bring him back into his body. 'And once you have an awareness of your body, you can start to build an awareness that I'm OK, I survived.' She continues, 'We talked a bit, through a translator, about things he could do to help him cope. We didn't talk about what had happened, or the loss of his son. There is a place for that – and maybe one day he can go through that in therapy if he wants to, but that's not what this is about.' She pauses. 'At the end, he said, "I have hope now."' These small epiphanies are often all Lisa sees. The results, she says, are rarely as dramatic as Peter Levine's patient escaping the tiger, and once a patient starts to feel a little better, it can be hard to persuade them to come back for a second session, making it difficult to measure progress. But she intuitively feels that helping people to become aware of their physical bodies is far more useful than talking – even if she doesn't have the science to back it up.

'The trouble is,' she admits, 'we don't really have an evidence base for this yet.'

As I leave, Lisa promises that I can come with her team on their next trip into the mountains in a few weeks' time, to see SE for myself. But the bad weather doesn't lift, so we never make it.

Leaving Nepal, I am frustrated that I never got to see somatic experiencing in action. On paper, I can't help but think it sounds very simplistic; and I can't really fathom how running away from an imaginary tiger could cure years of crippling anxiety. Of course, I understand that having a felt sense of safety is important – and that being held, or wrapped in a warm blanket, could help in the immediate aftermath of disaster. But I can't quite make the leap from this to the idea of physically shaking anxiety from the body.

Although the finer details of somatic experiencing may have escaped me, it still feels right that there are times when talking is not enough. If the language centre of the brain physically shuts down during extreme trauma, then of course talking about these memories wouldn't help, as they are cut off from language – beyond it. I know from my own experience of coming out that telling stories can give you a sense of control, and that it is therapeutic to arrange events into a neat and chronological order, with a beginning, middle and end. But there is a point at which this stops working, and there was always a central element of the experience that existed beyond language – a deep hurt and sadness that I never quite managed to articulate.

And so, in the end the stories became a defence, a way of

explaining and entertaining everyone else, that took me further from myself. Perhaps all I really needed was to be held, and to have a visceral, felt sensation of safety – like the headmaster when he was finally able to feel his feet again. And if Lisa is right, then that healing could only have come from the body, from silence.

Sitting in the airport in Kathmandu, I realise that in the weeks after coming out I *did* go in search of silence. I signed up to a silent retreat in the Trossachs and took a step back from the world. Perhaps I intuited that in silence I could find a source of healing and change – and so after the telling and re-telling of the kiss and the Thorong La I ran away to Scotland, as I simply couldn't face any more words.

PART FOUR

SILENCE

SCOTLAND

I REMEMBER STANDING AT STIRLING bus station between the
grey of the tarmac, the buildings and the sky. The world mono-
chrome, the air pithy with drizzle. There was still an hour before
my bus, so I took the escalator into the shopping centre, still
carrying my backpack. It had been two weeks since I had come
out, and I had left it all behind to be alone.

I had booked a few weeks off work as I was meant to be going
on holiday with my friend from Nepal, but after the kiss communication between us had broken down – and a holiday was out
of the question. Heartlessly, perhaps, I told her I didn't want to
see her. I had to work through the complicated morass of feelings on my own. Like George Oppen, I needed to hold the
thousand threads in my hand and see the single thing.[1]

I had started going to a Buddhist centre in London at lunchtime to meditate. It offered a space in those fraught days: half
an hour of sitting in silence, followed by tea and biscuits. They
would hand out leaflets about Buddhist retreat centres, along
with the digestives. A retreat, they suggested, would be a

chance to deepen our fledgling practice and 'investigate our experience'.

The idea of retreat sounded perfect. To run away, turn my back on the world and disappear for a while. It was the oldest strategy – the way I had survived at school – and now it was calling me back. I longed to slip into the anonymity of silence for a few days. I didn't really know what a retreat would involve. Maybe that's why I picked a place I knew. It was billed as a hillwalking retreat. Something had cleared, and crystallised, in the course of walking in Nepal. Waking up in the blue dawn, eating battered bread and jam from metal plates, fingers greasy, and then walking until the next meal. As the Romantic poets intuited, there is something about forward motion outside that stirs creativity; letting your brain look at things in a different way, while also allowing the sediment to settle. I wanted to be surrounded by the speechless Sublime. I hoped that a few days' walking in the Scottish Highlands would help me make sense of the preceding weeks. So much had been said, the story repeated over and again: crossing the Thorong La, the shape of my friend's dress, and mumbling the mantra 'I like women' over and over until the words didn't make sense.

The shopping centre in Stirling was striplight-bright, peopled with puffy flesh, tattoos and McFlurrys. Someone was shouting. I remembered Joan Didion writing that in the immediate aftermath of grief people look like they have been flayed – the outer layer peeled off, all offal, heart hanging out.[2] I felt like that. Not quite myself. Striding with an astronaut's gait in my walking boots on the polished lino floors of the shopping mall. I made endless circles looking for an ATM. I didn't know if there would be cash machines where I was going.

Back at the bus stand, cash in hand, a small woman with an elfin haircut and new hiking boots boarded the bus ahead of me. She was cowed, crustacean-like by her backpack. I wondered if we were going to the same place – but I didn't ask. We boarded the bus in companionable silence and watched the rain, as we headed west into the wet.

I had been this way before – for my twenty-first birthday we hired a minibus and drove up to the Highlands with twenty people on board. And the following summer I went wild camping in West Scotland with my ex-boyfriend. I remember watching the slow circle of a basking shark, as it siphoned the krill from the surface of the water, and carrying an air mattress down to the beach below. There was another summer too when I drove to look at the view with three friends. We watched the horizon through the sluiced windscreen like pensioners, warming our fingers around a thermos of tea. I felt at home. There is a Swedish word we don't really have in English – *trivs* – to thrive, to feel at home: '*jag trivs här*'. I thrived here, like moss on grey stone.

The Buddhist retreat was held in a converted hotel – a white-washed building on the shores of a loch. It was said to be fairyland, as in the seventeenth century the local vicar had been spirited away to the underground world of imps and goblins. He had written a book about 'the secret commonwealth of elves, fairies and fauns' and it was said the fairies stole him away on an afternoon walk, as revenge for exposing their secrets.[3] The miasma between this world and the next was porous here. It was easy to fall through.

When I arrived, language too was made strange. The Scottish retreat leaders used words I had not heard for a long time; ben, burn and lochan. I had not expected it to be so beautiful, so demonstrably alive. Everything seemed in flux; swallows swooped down and then back to roost under the eaves, never landing, and whorls of cloud moved across the fir forest on the other side of the loch. The bracken unfurled baby-fingered fronds in the wet of the morning. And the unexpected smell of coconut rose from the tight yellow-budded gorse.

Silence here was drip-fed. In hindsight, it reminds me of the procedure during somatic experiencing, where experience is 'titrated', so that the person being treated is led towards the powerful memories and then pulled back again to the safety of the present day.[4] We were told there would be silence overnight, and that the amount of silence would increase in increments each day, culminating in four days of silence at the heart of the retreat. I had never spent that long without speaking to anyone, and I was suddenly nervous. But there was nothing I could do; I had no car to drive away. And no buses came down that way. Everyone else seemed so at home; many were seasoned meditators who had been here before. They knew where to find the teabags and the custard creams. I felt like a fraud. I knew almost nothing about Buddhism and had never been on a retreat before. I was just someone drawn to spending time without talking.

Meals were communal, cooked and consumed together. We had to take turns at preparing food in the industrial kitchen, and as I reached the length of my arm inside the oversized cooking pots to peel away strings of rubbery porridge, I was reminded of my time at Cloyne Court, the student cooperative in California, where I had last cooked in a kitchen of this scale. It's funny how hard it is to see the thing itself without searching for a metaphor – or just the object, as Oppen would say. In these new surroundings I needed comparison for anything to make sense.

On the first night we ate greedily, and then retired to bed in silence. This first dose of silence felt artificial. I was sharing a room with two other women and as we moved towards bed we whispered theatrically, 'I'm done in the bathroom', or 'Sleep well'. Our actions were cartoonish in the proscribed stillness. It was the first time I had fallen asleep in a dormitory since school. The three single beds had matching cotton duvet covers, and I lay still as my roommates' breathing settled into sleep. This high in the northern hemisphere it stays bright late into the night, and I couldn't sleep. Blue slats of light fell across the dormitory floor from between the parted curtains, and I could hear the sound of moving water from the burn running down the hills to the dark loch below.

The following day we were awoken by the 6.30 a.m. rising bell. We meditated in silence in the morning for an hour, slathering ourselves with Skin So Soft, a scented moisturiser that is given to the American army as it keeps the midges at bay. I sat at the back of the shrine room, hoping no one would notice me. The room was a former outbuilding of the hotel, with a polished wooden floor and a small effigy of the Buddha at the front. The shrine was decorated with feathers, rocks and a bird's nest – cairns – things found and brought as offerings to the divine. Everyone arranged themselves on cushions or chairs, swaddling themselves in blankets, as we settled into stillness. From my place at the back of the room it felt as though the edges of the other people had begun to blur; all the others wore a retreat uniform of tracksuit bottoms or leggings, and thick socks. It was becoming harder to tell us apart.

At that first breakfast the forced hilarity of the silence continued: we raised our eyebrows to indicate that we needed the toast, and whispered theatrically for the peanut butter. After the early start, and an hour sitting in the chill of the morning, we ate ravenously. And in the silence, the taste of food was heightened. This was my first intimation of how other senses start to compensate when speech is withdrawn – perhaps just as the hearing of the blind is made more sensitive in the absence of sight. I could feel the oil of the peanut butter on my palate, the hard crusts of toast; the heat of the cinnamon and the earthiness of the seeds in the porridge.

The silence was gradually increased – at first just overnight – then stretching until lunch the following day, and within a few days we had attained 'full' silence. We were encouraged to leave notes on a message board for the retreat leaders if we felt we needed help, but otherwise we were left to our own devices. The days were broken down into a period of meditation before breakfast, then a period of teaching or a walk into the hills, then more meditation in the afternoon, dinner and bed. I felt a very visceral relief at the sense of order. It was strangely soothing having somewhere we had to be, whether that was chopping vegetables, scrubbing pots, helping in the garden, meditating or making packed lunches for the walk.

Thanks to the timetable, pinned to the communal notice board, I knew what everyone else was doing almost all of the time. It felt strange not explaining the turmoil of the previous weeks. In the silence there was no chance to tell stories, or explain who I was. This hiatus was a relief after the relentless dialogue of coming out. I sank into the silence, grateful for an end to the perpetual telling. After a few days, I began to notice that the way I interacted with other people had also shifted, as there was much less chance to look for validation – the social approval that dictates so much of what we do. In the early evenings I loved to sit in the reading room, watching the swallows dip and dive towards the lawn as the light faded. But whereas before I would have asked, 'Can I sit here?' or 'Is it OK if I turn the light on?', in the silence there was no opportunity to look for these small nods of approval, and so I stopped asking. They were such simple things – to sit on the sofa, or to take the last biscuit – but it felt strange to exist without the verbal tics of validation.

And without the anxiety of needing approval, I found my attention span began to stretch. I could read for hours at a time. Or sit and watch the movement of clouds across the horizon. Or write. And I did. I charted every bubbling emotion: the richness of the peanut butter in the morning, the calm as I read, and the growing sense of gratitude for the silence, for not having to justify myself or be good enough, or check if everyone was

OK. Looking back at the diaries of that week, I see that as the silence settled, I became enraptured with the countryside. I would walk along the loch and stop to touch the foxgloves, or the wet water-leaching bark. On sunny afternoons I would lie on a bench in the garden watching hard green cherries ripening in the sun, luxuriating in the warmth of the wood against my spine. Without words, or the need to seek approval, there was a sense of visceral and deep joy I had never experienced before. While on retreat I read Sara Maitland's astounding *Book of Silence*, which explained that my observations – heightened sensations, a sense of joy and greater calm – are all well-documented effects of silence, observed from the days of the Desert Fathers onwards.[5] I had never been in communal silence like this. I just knew there was a child-like delight in the purple of the foxgloves, or seeing a hare in the path – and having no one to tell I had seen it. And without the telling, the world seemed both more unreal and miraculous.

And as my attention stilled, my mind turned inwards too; so when I admired the dead red of the geraniums on the window-sill, I found bits of poetry bubbling up: T. S. Eliot's 'Midnight shakes the memory / As a madman shakes a dead geranium'; Sylvia Plath's tulips, the 'dozen red lead sinkers', too bright for her hospital room – the poems I had learnt in school. And alongside the poetry there were the words of hymns: 'He who would valiant be 'gainst all disaster, let him in constancy follow the Master', drumming around in circles as I did the washing up, dredged from the depths of memory by the potent mix of silence and the echo of the school environment – the dormitories, the lack of control or individuality – as we sat down to dinner in our uniform tracksuits. But in many ways the silence here felt like the opposite of the silence in the boot room: the lonely, covert, shameful silence of not having anything to say. This felt expansive; and as it was communal, a ritual practice that everyone was partaking in, I was not anxious about not saying anything. This wasn't billed as an ideal first retreat. Six hours of meditation a day and several days of complete silence. But I thrived – *trivs*. Maybe the days of silence in my youth had been training for this.

And then on the third night something became unhinged. It was the final meditation of the day and we were taught a mantra to repeat. It was the song of Green Tara, who I later learnt was a Bodhisattva – or enlightened being – who is said to embody compassion. We were singing to try and invoke this spirit of kindness. I had never experienced Buddhist ritual before and was sceptical of the murmuring in Pali, as it felt akin to reading out a Catholic catechism, when no one really knows what they are saying. But something strange happened. I began to cry – without being aware of feeling sad, or thinking about anything in particular – and I was unable to stop. I wiped hot tears onto my jeans and the blanket around my waist. I was glad I was at the back of the room, unobserved by the others. And as they rose to make offerings to the Buddha statue, I stood and walked out of the shrine room. Perhaps it was the energy of singing into the silence, after days of not speaking, or saying words I didn't understand, so that logic and cognition were sidelined – but something had been released.

By the loch I could still hear a murmur of faint singing, and the grass was wet against my flip flops. A few prayer flags, whitened in the sun, were strung like spider webs through the branches of a tree. As the singing stopped, it was silent apart from fish belly-flopping out of the water. I would hear the splash, but never quite saw them. I cried in a way I could not remember having done before: hands wet against my face, body doubled over. I had the sense of physically coming apart, and had no doubt that the silence had undone me.

So many people had asked if it felt like a weight was lifted when I came out, but if anything it felt like a loss. The loss of an imagined future, the loss of a friendship, the loss of the fixed and solid knowledge of who I was, and the losses of the past. I cried for the fifteen-year-old who didn't look to be loved back. For the disappointment of my parents. For not knowing what I was going to do when I got home. When it was over, I went back to the dormitories and slept like a child in the single bed with the cotton duvet. I didn't hear the others coming back from meditation.

I later learnt that among retreat leaders there is a phrase for this phenomenon: 'teary Tuesday'. It is so called as it is almost inevitable that after a few days of silence, buried emotions will reveal themselves. I didn't know this at the time – but I was beginning to understand that silence could be cathartic, a salve for buried hurt, just as it could be repressive.

On the train back to reality from Scotland the noise in the carriage swirled around me. I had a sense of being lost – detached somehow – watching the students laughing and drinking prosecco from plastic glasses, and the sticky-fingered children, pawing their parents. I did not feel part of the same world. I carried a little of the retreat silence with me, trying to delay my interaction with the world until the last possible moment.

SEARCHING FOR SILENCE

LOOKING BACK ON THE RETREAT, I find I still long for the stillness. And I begin to collect other people's experiences of silence as Eve had collected vaginas. I speak to the devout: a nun who talked about learning to walk quietly along the corridors of the convent; and a Buddhist teacher who tells me the thundering silence of the mountains gave her tinnitus. She had lived with the high-pitched ringing in her ears for eight years. Nothing made it better. In desperation she left the mountains and moved to London. There, between the hum of refrigerators and the moving traffic, she could ignore the constant tinnitus and come to something approaching silence. But 'true' silence is a loss she feels keenly. She apologises for her tears, as we speak. 'I'm sorry,' she says, 'I wasn't expecting to get so upset.' After meeting her, I speak to artists who spent time in silence, long before Marina Abramovic sat staring at the visitors in the gallery.[6] And I start to read more about silence – and what happens to the brain when there is nothing to say. I find that even in silence, the brain continues to 'hear' what is happening, as the auditory sensors keep on processing. So if you only think you hear a lyric to a song that's stopped playing, your brain thinks you are actually hearing it. Perhaps that was why the words of certain hymns kept coming back to me in Scotland – in the absence of sound, the brain will create its own.[7]

I learn that the World Health Organization estimates that noise contributes to millions of premature deaths in Western Europe each year[8] – and that, conversely, silence can be restorative. It is, as I intimated on retreat in Scotland, not simply an absence, but the site of growth and change. This was established accidentally in a study involving mice. Imke Kirste at Duke University Medical Center was researching the effects of sounds on the brains of mice in 2013. To do this, she played the mice different noises: music; baby mouse calls; white noise; and silence. Silence was intended to be the control aspect of the experiment, which she wasn't expecting to affect the brain. To her surprise, Imke found that two hours of exposure to silence a day prompted cell development in the hippocampus, the part of the brain related to the formation of memory involving the senses. It seems that in silence parts of the brain grow and re-form.[9] Puzzled, Imke speculated that this could be because the absence of sound is so unusual it prompted a higher level of alertness. But her study only related to mice – and I want to know more about how silence affects the human brain.

It isn't just silence I want. I crave what I had tasted on the retreat: a space where people come together with the explicit intention of not saying anything; a communal, curated silence. Somehow that shared space felt like the opposite of the quiet of my youth. I long for the tranquillity I had experienced in Scotland – where not speaking was a positive quality, something with an innate value – to be sought in and of itself.

In Scotland I had glimpsed for the first time that silence could provide a sense of community. And so I begin contacting monasteries and convents – and content myself with the silence of the library as I wait for their replies. The silence within the British Library's reading rooms is the closest I can get to a cloister. It feels like a living silence, built through joint effort and quiet industry. And I withdraw from the world as I write. I stop seeing friends and sink into the silence of the reading room, with its green leather desks and soft lighting.

I walk past the Friends' Meeting House on the Euston Road, on my way to the library, every day, but know very little about the Quakers, other than the fact that they practise in silence and are pacifists. I had heard apocryphal tales about them driving ambulances during the Second World War, as they refused to fight. So I decide to find out more about their brand of silence, and whether it is similar to the sense of community I had discovered in Scotland.[10]

When I arrive at the Sunday Meeting for Worship, the chairs are arranged in a series of circles, shell-like, with a small pile of bibles and a modest vase of flowers at the centre. The service begins as soon as the first person sits down, so when I walk in, a few minutes before the official start time, it is already in session. The idea of coming together for worship in silence in this way, I learn later, is rooted in the belief that every person has the capacity for direct communion with God, and therefore there is no need for priests or a set liturgy. All that is required is to sit and wait for direct insight into the nature of the divine.

It is a mixed congregation. A woman with bright pink hair pulls the focus to the front row as she cries soundlessly throughout most of the meeting, dabbing her eyes with a tissue and crossing and recrossing her legs. Older men sit hunched against sticks, hand over hand. It is hard to get a sense of these people, as silence irons out the creases and differences between us. There are those who look almost beatific – hands in laps, eyes closed, waiting for the spirit.

For the first half-hour we sit in settled silence. No one fidgets or checks their phones. And after a few minutes I feel the familiar fluidity of not being able to imagine where the edges of my body are once I close my eyes. A phrase they used a lot in Scotland about dropping down into the silence keeps coming to mind. And the silence seems to deepen with the passing time. I like that we can open our eyes and look at each other if we want, and that there isn't a pose we are meant to be in, like the set meditation posture on a pillow. We are simply required to be in the room, with an awareness of each other. Sitting quietly, without particular purpose. It is a pleasing change from the relentless counting and marking of breath on meditation retreats. The silence feels creative, alive; it is almost like being in a choir, each contributing to the absence of sound around us, and in so doing making it better for everyone. We are both creating and curating the stillness of the room.

But it is not a 'true' silence: the sounds of the world float around us. The floor vibrates with the shouts of a group of

Seventh-day Adventists who are using the room below, and there is the ceaseless grumble of the buses on the Euston Road. People come and go, shuffling with their coats and bags as they find or leave their place in the circle. After half an hour an elderly man gets to his feet, levering himself up on his cane. He speaks without embellishment, about the immigrants in Calais. It is the eve of a ferocious storm, he says, and surely there is a need to protect the more vulnerable. His voice sinks away as quickly as it had come. No one replies. It is strange to crowbar speech away from conversation. This is intrinsically different to the silence I had experienced in Scotland. It is a speaking into the silence: sound and its absence working together, like the word of God in the desert. Or something near the benevolent darkness of Samaritans; the sense of a listening room. And of course there is no answer to the plight of the refugees – the chaos and privation of young men waiting by the roundabouts of Northern France in the rain to try and jump under a lorry. Or at least there is no answer that could be reached in that room. Answering the man's question with silence feels more exploratory – and in many ways more sincere. It is refreshing to raise a problem and then let it sit in messy totality, rather than trying to come up with a response. A more authentic form of communication perhaps.

Twenty minutes later, a woman at the side of the room stands. She thanks the man – always using the non-differentiating moniker, 'friend' – and reflects on how she had worked in the 'Jungle' in Calais a few years ago, and how it had had a profound effect upon her. After another few minutes of silence an elderly woman stands, turning the rings on her fingers over and over. Her hands look swollen with arthritis, somehow too big for her wrists. There is a sense of confession in her words. She tells us that she has decided not to join a trip going to Calais as she is worried by the impending bad weather. We do not tell her not to worry. Her guilt sits in the silence with us all. Raising the complicated and messy – from international geopolitics, to personal conflicts – and not looking for answers, feels incredibly refreshing. The little bubbles of speech feel like the movements of a concerto: they speak to each other, but can stand alone, unlike a line of conversation, which is always contingent on what comes next.

Sitting in the silence after speech, I am reminded of an experiment I have read about, which looked at what silence does to the brain. It was conducted by a scientist called Bernardi, who studied people's responses to listening to music. He found the impact of listening to the music could be mapped in the body in differences in blood pressure or circulation, and generally resulted in states of arousal. But the most striking effect occurred between musical tracks, for he discovered that randomly inserted stretches of silence within a piece of music had a far more relaxing effect on the body than a relaxing piece of music; the heart slowed and blood pressure fell. What is interesting is that for the silence to have this effect it had to come within the music itself, as a random interruption – rather than during the silence at the start of the experiment. There is, it seems, something about silence after sound that has a profound effect upon the body.[11] And it was something about the unexpected juxtaposition of speech and silence at the meeting that I found most striking: somehow it changed the meaning of both.

The meeting ends with an invitation for the newcomers to stand and introduce themselves. I cringe, and look first at the floor and then my phone, and as soon as the other worshippers stand for tea and coffee, I move quickly down three flights of stairs and out into the central London traffic. I am a silence tourist – testing the waters, but not yet ready to admit I am here. But the meeting has deepened my sense that silence can be a positive quality, worth cultivating. I have a sense I will be back.

The idea of gravitating towards silence, as a positive quality, reminds me of an advertising campaign launched several years ago in Finland. It was aimed at the Asian market and tried to lure holiday-makers to the Nordic countries based on the fact that they were somewhere you could enjoy some peace and quiet. The slogan was 'Silence Please'.[12] The marketeers understood that silence was not simply an absence of a sound, but a commodity to be monetised: a golden egg on the wooded hills and trails and beside the vast lakes.

My extended family are Finnish, so I know that silence runs deeper than the open spaces of the countryside. At first I thought it was just the language barrier that caused the gaping holes in conversation. I would try and make small talk and it would fall entirely flat. I couldn't understand what was happening, as my relatives all spoke perfect English. 'Maybe you need to translate?' I would say to my partner. And when she did, they would smile at me confusedly. 'Yes,' they would say and nod. My partner later explained to me that small talk just doesn't exist in the same way in Finland. The idea of saying words simply to fill silence makes no sense there. According to anthropologist Michael Berry, Finnish silence can be traced to the country's relatively late industrialisation. He points out that Finnish urbanisation only took place around half a century ago. Before then, small talk was unnecessary – it was more essential to find food to put on the table.[13] Like the ice fishers in the Appalachian mountains whose children stopped speaking at school, it seems silence is culturally constructed. In Finland the pauses are an intrinsic part of conversation – not something to be avoided.

But as I discovered while trying to make small talk in Helsinki, if someone doesn't make conversation in the way you are expecting, it can provoke strong reactions, and I felt stupid when I found that I was on the outside of the conversational dance.

DEEP DIVE

'PEOPLE CAN HAVE A WHOLE host of reactions to silence,' Karin says, 'some people get very angry if you don't reply.'

Karin made the national press when she spent six months living in silence, on the eve of the millenium. She started the silence as an art project, and I found out about her experiment in old clippings from *The Mirror*.[14] As I read the pages of microfiche, I am astounded that an art student's silence could have made the national tabloids. I wanted to speak to her, to know how the world reacted to someone who had chosen to take a step back – as I had done as a child so many years ago.

We manage to speak one morning, after she has dropped her kids off at school. She now lives in the West Country, and is immediately self-deprecating when I mention the newspaper clippings. She laughs, 'Well, I went on to have a very normal life, I suppose.' She pauses. 'But it did feel like a very urgent thing at the time. It was just something I needed to do.'

She tells me she was a fledgling artist when she began her silence, and just felt a strong urge to 'go on retreat', as she was feeling 'fractured'. 'I was probably depressed at the time,' she says, 'although I don't like that label.' She believes this sense of fracturing and depression came from witnessing society's disregard for the environment. She tells me that as a child she spent a lot of time at sea and was raised by semi-nomadic parents. 'I think I almost saw the sea as a parent, in a way,' she says, and so the pollution of the oceans and the destruction of the ozone layer were wounds she felt keenly. She describes her silence as an experiment in communication, as she would still write notes if she needed to say anything. But she knew she needed to stop talking for a while. 'I saw the silence as a cocoon,' she explains, a warm and healing space, in which to retreat from the world.

This silence had to be carefully curated. Karin had chosen to communicate using only the written word during the experiment, and so, in the days and weeks before the silence began, she told her friends and family what she was planning to do, and even went to the local shops to explain that she would be using a notepad and pen to communicate for the next six months. She made sacrifices in order to do this, like a nun who gives up worldly goods and the delights of the flesh on entering her order. 'It was a personal calling that I felt I had to respond to quite fast,' she says. She paid for her time in silence by living off her credit cards, as it would have been impossible to have held down a job, and she didn't want to wait for Arts Council funding. But when she began the silence she was in a relationship, they soon broke up as it was simply not possible to maintain that level of intimacy without speech. 'We were already drifting apart, to be honest,' she says, 'and it became clear that it wasn't possible during something like that.' She pauses. 'I don't think it would have been desirable for me either, as it would have stopped me from going deeper. It was like a deep dive.'

As she describes her 'deep dive', I am struck by the similarities between her silence and the speechlessness of selective mutism. The silence was, she recalls, an 'isolating' time, as she was always having to deal with other people's reactions to the fact she wasn't speaking. 'You can blend in,' she says, 'until someone speaks to you, and then it's awkward when someone says "Hello" and you don't answer.' As a result, she initially withdrew from the world as it was too difficult to be in social situations without speaking. She found some people would get angry. 'Their reactions often told you more about them than me,' she says, but nonetheless it was not always easy to field their frustration with her experiment in communication. As she talks, I recall the stories of teachers berating the selectively mute and silent child, and my own frustrations filming at WeSpeak, watching the faltering stop start of conversation with the kids, and not being able to build a relationship with them. And yet, even with these hardships, Karin found not speaking to be addictive – a habit that was hard to break. The silence was meant to be for three months, but it spread into six. Thanks to her careful preparation, the world accommodated her, and so there was no incentive to change.

But her silence was different to that of a selectively mute child in one crucial aspect: it was chosen. And perhaps because of this element of choice, she found it to be an enriching experience, an experiment in exactly what needs to be said, rather than 'true silence'. As she explains: 'You can't do small talk in writing, if you're going to write something down it has to be worth the time and the energy, so generally speaking the things that I shared felt more important. I felt that I had a lot of deep connection and conversations with people during that time,' even though those conversations were written down rather than spoken. And having this written dialogue was in a sense the point of the experiment. 'That was my interest as an artist,' she says, 'it was provoking people to think about choice and communication.'

But something else happened during Karin's silence. In the 'deep dive', her sense of self started to metamorphose. 'I wasn't the same person when I came out of the silence as when I went in,' she says. 'Silence is very depersonalising – it takes you out of your personal individual self.' She thinks this is because so much of our sense of who we are is bound up in language and speech. We are always expressing opinions, or forming new connections with people by talking, and it is this which marks us out as a person. 'It really was quite strange to hear my voice after all those months,' she says. 'It was very strange, because in a sense your separate self is so bound up with your speaking voice. In silence you feel less separated – your sense of self is very different. What going into deep silence allows is for you to sit with reality in a very different way. You're not constantly referring to the codes of language.' And without language she had a more immediate experience of the world. 'I could see things differently,' she says. 'It is almost like pulling back from culture and getting a bird's eye view that you just don't see when you're in the middle of engaging with everyone all the time. I had the sense of everything being connected and interconnected.'

I have some sense of what she means by this. In the course of the retreat in Scotland I found that in many ways it was easier to forge connections with people without speaking. There was no opportunity to find out that you disagreed politically with someone, or didn't share the same sense of humour. Somehow, stripping away conversation gave a greater sense of shared humanity. And without speech my sense of self also felt shaky. It was strange not being able to draw the outlines of my being by telling people I was a journalist. No one could be impressed by the fact I had recently been filming in Afghanistan. And conversely I couldn't look for reassurance by saying it was my first retreat, and that I didn't really know what I was doing. Without the stories we wrap around ourselves, it was harder to find the edges of myself.

Karin says that if she went into silence again she wouldn't write things down, as with hindsight she thinks the written language 'contaminated' the silence. She laughs, 'It sounds strange to say that, but words are just symbols. It is a way of describing – it is not the thing itself.' Language got in the way of the sense of connection she felt to the world. As she explains, 'Silence is being able to be with existence itself without any of the codes we weave around it.'

I am staggered by this – as it is an almost verbatim summary of Oppen's understanding of language. He said, time and again, that words were not transparent. They got in the way. And the fact that they came between the viewer and the experience in some ways made them 'heartless'.[15] They were the only tools he had – and yet they were broken. Writing about the world was, for Oppen, like a child scooping up the water in a lake to try and catch their reflection. Perhaps this explains the poet's fascination with silence, for if words are always getting in the way, then silence offers the chance of deeper communion.

The idea that silence could both unhinge your stable sense of self, and allow a closer communion with the world, is compelling. After talking to Karin, I begin to wonder what it would be like to go back into silence – to see what it feels like to slip into the abyss for a second time. I am greedy for the emptiness.

And so, almost four years to the day from that wet summer morning in Stirling, I go back to the retreat centre in Scotland. It is strange to return. Like coming home to family at Christmas, going back to the same place seems to concertina time. But the weather is darker this time, not the bright brilliant sunshine on the loch and cherries in the sun, but damp – in the air, the curtains, the grass. I cannot walk barefoot on the lawn, as the peat-brown water leaches up underfoot. And I shuffle awkwardly between the buildings in flip-flops and socks, the dark dots of midges dead on my skin.

For the first time the silence feels debilitating. I am bored and restless, and start taking long walks away from the retreat centre. On the second day, as I walk back from the loch, I see an injured sheep by the side of the road, its eyes rolling back in its head. It feels heartless, somehow, to meet its suffering in silence. I want to tell someone, to gather help. The note I leave on the communal notice board asking if the retreat leaders could contact the local farmer feels utterly inadequate. Like ululating women at a funeral, its suffering demands sound.

I find it is also harder to share humour in silence, as it seems to deaden both extremes of the emotional spectrum. I am standing by the loch one afternoon when a woman walks alongside me, pulls off her skirt and walks naked into the water. I want someone to turn to and ask, 'Did you see that?' Or to talk through the correct course of action when a stranger gets naked beside you – is it better to back away, as if nothing has happened, or to keep watching, as if it's no big deal? I watch the white cheeks bobbing at the surface. Shock and humour are emotions that must be shared – they just don't work in a vacuum. And if you can't share a joke, then one of the richest aspects of human experience is lost.

This emotional flattening reminds me of a passage in *A Book of Silence* where Sara Maitland describes a condition known as accidie, a form of listlessness and depression which is caused by prolonged periods in silence. It comes from the Greek *a-kedos*, meaning 'not caring', and is characterised by a total lack of interest in life.[16] The accidie sufferer will find it difficult to get up in the morning, or to move from staring out the window. Life becomes colourless, as accidie is, according to Maitland, 'an overwhelming sense of blankness and a restless and dissatisfied boredom'. It was, she writes, a common affliction among silent monastic orders and is directly related to extended periods without speaking. The only way to treat accidie is by the imposition of strict routine and discipline, without which you simply fall into torpor. It had never occured to me before that the endless timetabling on the retreat could be a way of stopping us from dropping into apathy. But suddenly the endless rounds of cooking, meditation, Buddhist instruction and meals seem a necessary antidote to the freeform whorl of silence. As I lie on my bed one drizzly afternoon, staring listlessly towards the loch, listening to the hand bell being rung to call us to dinner, it occurs to me that silence could be dangerous. It would be all too easy to simply lie here, staring into space. For the first time I realise the silence has to be held in check, divided into manage-able portions of work or meditation, to make it bearable. In unlimited silence, I could see how you could start to disappear.

And just as I am starting to think about the potentially deadening, destabilising nature of silence, my roommate will not stop speaking. She says she is new to meditation, and I don't think she had realised that so much of the week would be spent in silence. I feel for her on one level. But on another it is infu-riating, as she stops me from being quiet. Silence, I realise, has to be a joint effort, like conversation. The strain of not speaking seems to leave her jumpy and scattered. Whenever we are in the room together, she tries to engage me in conversation – mouthing her words in an exaggerated stage whisper. She begins narrating what is happening. 'I'm off to meditation now,' she whispers, 'are you coming? Oh, are you sleeping? Do you want anything? I'm going downstairs.' Every movement needs to be validated by speech. And as the days go on, she becomes angry. Nothing is clear, she says, fighting back the tears. The retreat leaders don't explain well enough to her what is happening. The silence is disempowering and scary – she can't navigate it. In the end, she leaves. She packs up and drives away after three days. The retreat leaders keep her place in the shrine room – an empty pillow and folded blanket a reminder of her absence.

Sitting looking at her empty place, it seems an apt emblem for the difficult nature of silence, which is, I am beginning to understand, something that needs to be bounded and controlled by timetables and hand bells. And it can deaden the extremes of human emotion and be deeply uncomfortable, prompting an almost allergic reaction in the uninitiated.

I come away from the retreat with a newfound respect for silence. And I want to know how people who spend months or even years living without speaking cope with the absence of language. Do they drop into the torpor of accidie, or feel their sense of self becoming unhinged? I am finally starting to get some responses to the emails I had sent to various silent religious orders. And so I arrange to pay one of them a visit.

GOING MAD

THE NUNS OF TYBURN CONVENT are an entirely silent order in the heart of central London. The entrance to the convent is on the Bayswater Road, as you go towards west London. It was a site of executions as late as the eighteenth century and it was here that Catholic martyrs were hanged at the notorious Tyburn Tree.[17] The convent looks out over Hyde Park, by Speakers' Corner, the site of so much noise. The Tyburn sisters have renounced almost all contact with the world. They leave the cloisters only for medical appointments, to meet a sister arriving at the airport from another convent, or to vote. Their lives are dedicated to prayer, and as such there is always one nun present in permanent supplication to the Virgin in the convent's chapel.

I am late. I run from the bus, looking for the front door. It isn't marked, but sits between the down-at-heel hotels and smart mansion blocks. Tourists walk past en route to Hyde Park and shoppers stagger by, laden with brown-paper Primark bags. Street artists have hung their wares against the park railings where the Tyburn Tree would once have stood. It is hard to imagine the martyrs turning by their necks here. I push open what I assume is the front door, and the silence hits me like the heat as you leave a plane: unexpected and arresting. A nun kneels in prayer. She doesn't move as the door opens. There is something staggering about her vulnerability – kneeling without locks on the door, in a chapel that opens directly onto the chaos of the Bayswater Road. The noise and fumes swell into the chapel. It is otherworldly; only the bright white of her habit is visible as my eyes adjust to the darkness. I stand for a second, watching. The rosary clicks. The motes drift in the light from the door. I want to stay, to sit in this silent space as she prays. But I am late, so I close the door and am back in the sound of the world.

The entrance to the convent is a few metres further down the road and opens onto a holding area. There are displays about the history of the convent and a glass cabinet containing trinkets made by the nuns – peg dollies and knitted angels.[18] After I ring the bell, the inner door is opened by a young woman in a dark habit.

'I've come to see Mother Hildegarde,' I say.

'Come this way.'

She leads me down a dimly lit corridor, our shoes squeaking on the lino floor. The smell of bleach on the wipe-clean surfaces immediately reminds me of school and the 'backstairs' that the girls could use which ran up to the 'dorms' from the 'house study' where we did our 'prep'. Everything had its own word; the tribal sense of belonging marked by a shared lexicon. The main carpeted stairs were for staff and sixth form only. The backstairs ran down towards the house kitchen with its blue lino floor, where we would hold birthday parties: eating chocolate spread out of the jar and loosening our ties to dance to Stereophonics.

I am led into a waiting room. A jug of water with a linen doily laid over the top and a plate of custard creams await me. The china is also the same issue as at school: off-green. Not quite a colour. The room is utilitarian: a rocking chair and a dresser with books about Catholicism, an unlit gas fire, a table and two other chairs. As I wait, I am struck again by the silence, and the energy, of people moving along the corridors without making noise. There is no murmur of voices. No footfall in the corridor. I presume the nuns must have rubber-soled shoes – like the baddies in the Secret Seven books.

When Mother Hildegarde arrives, she is not what I expected. She is a large Australian woman who starts telling me about silence before she has fully sat down, barely stopping to draw breath.

'So you want to know about silence?' she begins. 'Well, there are two types of silence, or there's two types of noise, I should say. The two types of noise you've got are outside noise and interior noise, so if you want to learn about silence you have to first cultivate the outside to be more silent, then you can cultivate the inside to be silent. For silence you need to curtail the outside, and what we do here is we only talk in places where we need to talk, we don't have general chitchat: "Oh, how are you, how are you going?"'

She finally pauses, to arrange herself on the chair, and looks longingly at the custard creams. Our conversation will continue in this vein for the next two and a half hours, in meandering streams of consciousness, punctuated by my occasional question. Part of her vocation within the convent is to talk to the media. Presumably she felt called to the role as she is gregarious, engaging and keen to chat – even when the dictaphone is off and my bag is packed, jacket on, ready to leave. I am reminded of the desperation of the elderly who would call Samaritans on a Sunday afternoon, eager to talk – needing the low-level human interaction when you have no one else to speak to.

When I say that she seems to miss chatting, she laughs. 'When I told my friends I was going to be nun, they all said, "Well, I have no doubt you're religious – but do you know in those places you have to keep quiet?"' She looks straight at me. 'And I said, "Well, you can learn" – and that's basically it, you learn to be quiet. I'm normally over-chatty, but when you are in the monastery you keep it down.' She laughs, 'But I'm a banger and a crasher, so I didn't find silence easy at first.'

She tells me she joined the order relatively late in life, when she was already in her thirties and things hadn't worked out quite as planned. She is intentionally vague, but tells me that she had realised her marriage was not working and that she had an increasing sense of religious calling. Her family had not understood her desire to enter silence and to leave her friends, her job, her home. 'I was in the process of saving for a deposit for a house,' she says, 'I had an excellent job, but this nun thing kept coming up.'

When she decided to join the religious order, she couldn't find the words to tell her parents in person. So she wrote them a letter – perhaps, as Karin discovered, there are some things that are better communicated in writing. 'I suppose writing the letter was a coward's way out,' she says. 'My dad didn't speak to me for two years – he swore at me, and said I was locking myself away in a prison.' But even though she was entering a largely silent order, she was told not to break contact with her family. 'My novice mistress said, "You must write to your father."' This was unusual, as the nuns are normally only allowed to send a certain number of letters per month, to keep the cost of postage down, in line with their vow of poverty. She was awed by the gesture. 'And I didn't really know what to talk about,' she says, 'but the novice mistress said, "Just write to him." So I just sent off these little cards, that said things like, "I love you dad" or "I hope to hear from you soon".' There is something so painful about throwing these words into the silence. And, as I imagine the novice nun writing her notelets of love, I am struck once again by the way silence is so often met with anger – like the kids with SM, or Karin and her handwritten cards.

Now Mother Hildegarde is only allowed to receive phone calls and visits once a month – although she tells me that she doesn't miss her family any more. There are so many unexpected echoes of school in the monastic life, and the monthly scheduled phone calls transport me back to the phone box in the boot room. I started boarding when I was fifteen, as I thought it would be easier to make friends. At that time, mobile phones were a rarity, so any contact with the outside world was conducted via the communal phone box. The walls were made of plywood, with coils of biro graffiti etched into them. You could hear everything that was being said. Everyone could sign up for a ten-minute slot on the phone each night, and the next person was usually waiting outside for their turn. The lack of privacy was corrosive. I found it almost impossible to have a normal conversation in a prearranged time slot. But for Mother Hildegarde, this is a sacrifice she was happy to make for the sake of her relationship with God.

The purpose of being in the silent order, she explains, is to allow the nuns to make space for God. And as such the silence is creative not nihilistic. 'One lady asked me if it was being totally empty, and I said no,' she says, 'I don't believe in that. You have to have room for you and God. You are who God created, you are His person, and you have to be who you are – you just need to tone it down a bit to allow space for Him.' She smiles. 'And if you do that, God will start showing you things.' Silence, for the sisters of Tyburn, gives insight into their true nature, and the world around them. And that is worth any amount of privation.

She explains that the silence is maintained through a series of checks and balances, including a ticket system, whereby a nun writes out a ticket if she is unwell or needs permission to leave the monastery for any reason. And within the walls, the silence is never absolute. The nuns are able to talk to each other during weekly 'recreation' sessions, and it is possible to request an 'auditorium' with a more senior 'mother' if you have problems. And despite the fact that the sisters spend most of their days in silence, she tells me there is a strong sense of community – and she repeatedly describes the convent as a family. Perhaps it is an apt comparison as so often families rub along on the assumption that not everything will be said.

I'm struck by the safety valves to keep the silence controlled – like the option of an auditorium or recreation – and I get the sense that silence is powerful, something to be monitored and limited. When I mention this, Mother Hildegarde tells me that when she joined the order the thing that worried her the most was that she had had counselling. She had a whole life that she was signing away, and was worried they might think she was not stable enough to enter the order, as the demands of the silent life are rigorous. And when she first joined, the silence was destabilising – she had visions. 'When I first entered,' she says, 'I nearly left because I kept getting these awful thoughts. There was rudeness, and rape and all sorts coming in – and I started thinking I'm not fit to be a nun.' But as she was on her way to see the novice mistress, to confess her terrifying visions, she realised where the images might have come from. In her previous life she had been a self-confessed 'movie buff', and she realised that in the silence, half-forgotten scenes from horror films were coming back to haunt her as otherworldly visions of rape and torture. 'I suddenly realised it was from the movie *Alien*,' she says, 'the rape things were coming out of the movies I had watched, and in the end all I had to do was identify which movie it was, and then I said "get out", and it stopped. It was no longer.'

Back in the sunshine I am aware of the pull of conversation – or rather of the fact that Mother Hildegarde just didn't want to stop talking. And I am also struck by the way silence percolates your experience, so that you can end up walking the lino corridors experiencing flashbacks of rapes you have seen on screen years before. As I board the bus home, it occurs to me that perhaps these frightening visions are not so surprising; in most major religious texts strange things happen in silence: the Devil appears to tempt Jesus in the emptiness of the desert; and the Buddha hears the voice of the demon Mara as he sits in silence under the Bodhi tree. There is something about surrendering yourself to silence that means you can't control what comes up.

But in all religions there is the impulse to go deeper – to disappear into the desert and sit with your experience in silence. I began to wonder what happens if you go into deep silence, without a community surrounding you, or even anyone to write notes to? What happens if you combine silence with solitude? I knew the Buddhists put a particular premium on being alone. When on retreat I had seen the little huts up the hill, with shadowy figures sitting outside watching the clouds, like the ghosts that come up on film – translucent echoes of people. No one spoke to them or interacted with them. They were, I was told, 'on solitary' – spending weeks or months in solitude and silence as part of their Buddhist practice. And I had heard that some will do much longer periods of solitude – supported by a community, but not part of it, so that food is provided for them, but not company. I was intrigued. If living in a silent community could drive you to the edge of insanity – plagued by visions of extra terrestrial rape – then what did spending nearly a year with only yourself for company do? I needed to go further into the real 'deep dive' of silence.

I meet Deva Mitra in a backroom of the London Buddhist Centre. The cup of tea before me is frothy with soya milk and entirely unappetising. Before our meeting I watched his teaching videos on YouTube, but in real life he looks smaller. His frame has been shrunk by months of cancer treatment. His hair, in a ponytail in the videos, has just started to grow back, prickled across his skull; and the edges of his body are hidden in clothes just a little too big now. I have arranged to speak to him, as before he became ill with prostate cancer he spent nine months living on solitary retreat. He understands the joys and perils of silence intimately.

The centre is running a respite morning for carers when I visit, and I can hear children somewhere above us. Outside there is the constant growl of traffic on the Roman road which runs out of London to Colchester, where the imperial armies once marched. I have been here a handful of times before. Just after coming out I went to a meditation group for bisexual women. We were told to walk around the room in silence and to feel our feet on the polished wooden floor; moving in slow circles, before the half-closed eyes of an enormous gilded Buddha.

Deva Mitra tells me that his name means 'friend of God' in Pali, the ancient Indian language spoken by the Buddha. The name was given to him when he was ordained as a Buddhist, and is, he tells me, intended both to sum up his qualities as a person and give him something to aspire to. He has been an ordained member of the Triratna Order for forty-five years.[19] Deva Mitra joined when he was in his early twenties. At the time he was a struggling actor, fresh from a trip trekking in Nepal. While there, he contracted pneumonia and ended up being treated in a Buddhist monastery, as he was too unwell to continue the ascent. 'I was struck by the kindness of the monks there,' he tells me. 'They didn't need to help us, but they did. And the more I watched them, the more I realised they had something that I didn't – and I wanted it.' Since then he has been practising and exploring the Buddhist path and, he explains to me, a crucial part of that is learning to sit with yourself in solitude.

He explains that solitary retreats are an essential part of the Buddhist tradition, as the Buddha encouraged his disciples to go and meditate on their own, away from the distractions of civilisation. The Buddha himself achieved enlightenment while sitting in silence under the Bodhi tree, and once enlightened the Buddha talked about silence as being 'Aryan' or 'noble', and advised his monks that unless they were engaged in discussion about the scriptures, they should remain mute. 'Silence is obviously very important,' Deva Mitra explains, 'because it throws you back on your own experience.' He pauses. 'So often we distract ourselves through conversation. And that's why so much conversation is really rather superficial, as we are seeking distraction from our immediate experience through talk.' This makes sense to me – I suppose it is the reason walking in the rain and complaining to a companion about how wet it is doesn't feel as soul-destroying as weathering the storm alone. Something about talking dilutes the immediacy of the experience. But at the same time, I am struck by the fact that rather than distractions, friends, family, work and idle pleasures like reading or cooking seem to be the very fabric of life itself. What is left if you remove all these 'distractions'? Deva Mitra was determined to find out.

Like Mother Hildegarde, he is keen to talk about his experiences in silence. He calls me back almost as soon as I have emailed to request an interview, and our conversation stretches until lunchtime. I get the sense that he wears the prolonged isolation like a veteran's scars. He jokes that the idea of spending nine months in silence first came up as a competition, as another Order member had just completed an eight-month solitary retreat – but I get the sense that it also came, as it did for me in Scotland, at a moment of crisis, a crossroads. On one of his YouTube talks about the retreat, he says that at the time he had nowhere to live, and his mother had just died. His responsibilities were gone, and he was cut adrift.

His retreat took place in the mountains of southern Spain, stretching from the short dark days of winter to the eventual light of May. He was supported by a Buddhist community, who would bring him a food parcel and other basic supplies every few weeks, but would not make direct contact with him. His hut had running water and a wood-burning stove for warmth. He brought a handful of books about Buddhist scripture to read, but would only allow himself forty minutes a day: twenty minutes at lunchtime, and another twenty minutes at the end of the day, so that he would not be distracted from his immediate experience. Other than that, he says, he 'did very little'. His days were divided up between a little light exercise, four periods of meditation, and fetching wood for the stove. Initially, he found the silence deeply pleasurable. 'I think silence is something which has a value of itself,' he says, 'a bit like love in a way. It's something which many people are frightened of, but if only you can relax into it it is so transformative, so enjoyable.'

But one afternoon, during the witching hour of 4 p.m., which the unemployed and idle know so well, when there is nothing left to do and the day is not quite over, he felt a sudden wave of fear. He went weak at the knees. Not unlike the first rush of love perhaps. 'My legs just went weak and shaky,' he says, 'it was this horrible sensation. I had expected it to start getting difficult, so in a way I wasn't surprised.' But his silent trials were only beginning.

A few months later, he was gathering wood in the late-afternoon sun. He had rigged a harness across his chest to allow him to pull large quantities of logs up to the hut, and as he braced himself against the load, he felt something give way. He stopped and pressed his hands to the spasm in his chest, and realised he had pulled an intercostal muscle, one of the ribbons of sinew running between his ribs. The pain wouldn't go away. Several weeks passed, and he couldn't shake the pulsating pain radiating from the damaged muscle. 'I knew I had simply pulled a muscle in my chest,' he says. 'I knew it wasn't that bad, but I couldn't get the idea out of my head that I had strained my heart.' And in the silence, with no one to speak to for reassurance, his grasp on reality began to slip. He thought he was dying. He would lie in bed at night, with anxiety churning through his body. 'This tremendous fear welled up,' he says, 'I really felt I was going mad.' The muscles in his thighs began to convulse and his 'guts were spinning'. His body was beyond his control. His muscles were locked in spasm and he vomited. He recalls lying on the bed, trying to get a handle on his physical symptoms and racing thoughts, and thinking, 'My mind has a will of its own, my body has a will of its own. How can I get beyond that? What can I do?'

In the end, the effects of the silence and solitude were so intense that he decided to break his retreat conditions and speak to someone in the outside world. He had brought an old phone with him, for use in emergencies, and he dialled a friend who was a doctor. With no control over his mind or body, he needed advice. More than that, he needed language, an anchor, something to hold onto; something to pull him away from the experience. The doctor listened carefully to his symptoms and reassured him that he was not having a heart attack – and the act of speaking to someone calmed him. Or perhaps the reality of being heard, of being recognised as a person, with human needs, was all he needed after months of ascetic isolation. He hung up the phone and collapsed into sleep.

But the strange symptoms continued, and he made several further phone calls. 'I really felt I was losing my mind,' he says, 'and knew I was in desperate danger of blowing a once-in-a-lifetime opportunity. So I made a decision. No more calls for outside help. Even if you think you're dying, you've just got to face death.' It was only then, having decided to face death, that his symptoms subsided. 'It's pretty tough medicine, solitude,' he says.

It is interesting that, like the nun plagued by visions of rape, it is only when Deva Mitra spoke to himself that the madness stopped. There is something about naming and addressing a sensation that makes it manageable, knowable, rather like Adam naming the world in Eden and claiming stewardship over the plants and animals. Language inevitably bestows some degree of control. Once he had regained mastery of his body and his thoughts, Deva Mitra began to consider what had happened. 'I suddenly thought, "Hang on a minute, if my mind had a will of its own and my body had a will of its own, then where did that idea come from? Where did the perception that my mind has a will of its own come from?"' He laughs at the slightly mind-bending idea of thinking about your own consciousness. His terrifying experiences, he tells me, unwittingly gave him some insight into the nature of being, which, from a Buddhist perspective, extends beyond a fixed and unified self. He believes his experiences in silence gave him a glimpse of a vast consciousness far beyond normal experience. Something beyond our thoughts and bodies. He pauses, leaning forward, 'Consciousness is enormous. But our experience of it is so limited, so it tends to be very narrow, we narrow it all down to me. But you get glimpses in solitude when that narrowness just begins to disintegrate and opens up into something much more vast.'

After we speak, I stay to attend the lunchtime meditation session. As I arrange myself on a stack of pillows, I can't quite get my head around the idea of the 'vastness of consciousness'. I suppose that's my enduring problem with Buddhism, that the idea of enlightenment or ever-expanding consciousness seems as unbelievable as an old man in the sky. But what does make total sense is that after prolonged silence and solitude you would feel you were going mad – and that your stable, solid sense of self would begin to disintegrate. In the end, Deva Mitra managed to still the terror, but to do that he had to prepare for the fact that he might actually be dying, and also make peace with the terrifying realisation that he had no control over his mind or body. He had forty-five years of experience of meditation. And silence still nearly broke him.

I open my eyes and look around the room. It is busy, on a random Monday lunchtime. There is a full gamut of ages and genders here. Some are lying on the floor, others perch on chairs, or are balanced, serene, on cushions. Many have brought their bags into the room with them, and sit with a purse or a phone beside them. Someone is shouting outside on the Roman road. I am surprised by how many people are here. Mindfulness and meditation are currently enjoying a renaissance – and are even taught in primary schools. They are offered on the NHS.[20] They are, we are told, a panacea – for stress, sadness, for life itself. I am surprised, looking around me, how many people are willing to try sitting in silence in the hope of inner peace. Deva Mitra made it clear that meditation is a confrontation with experience, and in the course of that confrontation you could encounter some pretty terrifying emotions. I wonder how many of these lunchtime meditators are aware of the potency of silence. How it can unhinge you. Maybe Deva Mitra was right in his description of silence as like love – tempting, intuitively right. But it can also so easily lead you down a rabbit hole, where nothing is as it seems.

THE DARK NIGHT

ONCE YOU START LOOKING INTO the darker side of silence, you soon end up in some strange corners of the internet. One evening I find myself on a forum dedicated to a phenomenon called 'the 'dark night'. I read message boards peopled with experiences of dissociation, panic and suicidal thoughts. The dark night seems to be a name given to the stranger, scarier experiences people have had during the silence of meditation, invoking the 'dark night of the soul' suffered by St John of the Cross. I read the experiences avidly – impressed by the fact that it does not seem to take nine months in silence for body and mind to fall apart. And it is here that I meet Anna. Like me, she is lurking on the message boards, looking for people who would speak to her about their experiences in silence.

'The dark night is when meditation goes wrong,' she tells me, over Skype from Australia a few days later. I long for the sun pouring into the room behind her. She is wearing a bikini under her shirt, and there is a little dog in the room. She is currently completing a research masters in dark-night experiences, and thinks the number of people having difficult experiences during meditation could be related to the way we understand meditation as a quick fix for stress. 'I think it's important to realise,' she says, 'that meditation in the West at the moment is basically conceptualised as stress reduction or relaxation, or a health-promoting technique. But in a religious context, meditation was not about stress relief. It was about becoming enlightened – it's realising the true nature of self and connecting with the divine.' She laughs. 'So that is not meant to be an easy path. Traditionally meditation was not something that every monk did.' And perhaps unsurprisingly, if this practice is open to the general public during drop-in sessions at lunchtime, scary things can start happening.

It was when Anna first started practising meditation herself that she had the first indication that prolonged periods in silence were not for everyone. She tells me she had been working in the corporate sector and took up meditation as a 'cool thing to do', and also as a form of stress relief. But even in the early sessions, as soon as she sat in silence her mind began to play tricks. 'I would get these terrible headaches,' she says, 'and I would see this bright purple light in the centre of my vision.' She began to feel increasingly disconnected from the world and describes one meditation session where 'everything fell away' and she had the sense that nothing existed apart from herself and the meditation teacher in the room. These feelings of dissociation persisted into her normal life. 'I was in a bookstore, and I had an overwhelming feeling of being disconnected from the world. It was like a magic eye puzzle; like I had seen the picture, and couldn't go back to seeing just the dots again.' In the weeks that followed, these dissociative experiences continued and she began feeling more and more disconnected from the world and eventually developed clinical depression.

Listening to her, I realise I might have been stupid to dive into that first silent retreat in Scotland without adequate preparation. Like Anna, I had never experienced prolonged silence before and had not read anything about Buddhism – I just knew I needed to be quiet. Anna was able to treat the depression with medication, but the dissociative experiences persisted – and sparked her interest in 'the dark night'. Looking back, she says she doesn't know if meditation was solely to blame for her depression. At the time her life was in freefall: her mother had just been diagnosed with cancer, her marriage had broken down and she had left her job. But it was meditation that she links to the feelings of depersonalisation and dissociation – of not being quite in the world. It sounds not unlike the children with SM, as life flows around them. And once these feelings of dissociation start, they are hard to shake off.

As she talks, I am reminded of a conversation I had with a psychologist called Miguel Farias in the course of my research. He set out to investigate if meditation could really change you – and emerged with a deep scepticism of much of the science behind mindfulness.[21] One of his theories is that we are just not suited to meditation in the modern age. 'Two hundred years ago,' he told me, 'the social structures and structures of meaning were clearly delineated. Now, we have insecure structures of work, and meaning and class and religion have all fallen down.'

He pauses. 'I think these contemplative methods were probably developed for people who had a much more robust sense of self – who knew where they stood.'

Perhaps it was spending time in silence with her experience that unbalanced Anna – or perhaps it was the ontological instability of everything else, with her family and relationships in flux. More likely, it was the complex interrelation of the two – something which would not have happened to the ascetics of the twelfth century. It is perhaps not silence itself that is dangerous, but the context in which it occurs.

Of course, most people practice meditation without any adverse reactions, but I soon find Anna is not alone in suffering some very strange experiences. Another, older woman tells me that she had started experimenting with Zen meditation at the onset of the menopause – and ended up hospitalised and psychotic.

Jane had been a yoga teacher for twenty years, but the hot flushes caused by the onset of the menopause meant it was increasingly difficult for her to practise. So she began looking to channel her energy into something else. Zen meditation fitted the bill – a particularly intense form of concentration, requiring practitioners to engage in free-form meditation, simply sitting with their experiences in silence, without mantras or breathing exercises to cling to. She found the practice deeply compelling and began attending Zen retreats. And it was on one of these retreats that things started to go wrong.

On the first night of the retreat, Jane tells me she felt her mind 'fizzing' and was unable to sleep. She lost her appetite and ate only bread and water for the week. She had never struggled with her mental health before, so she didn't realise that these were the first warning signs of a growing psychosis. Looking back, she can't say if it was definitely the meditation and time spent in silence that triggered this initial psychosis – but she thinks it made it more intense than it might have been otherwise. She tells me she was aware that her behaviour was unusual, so asked the retreat leader about it and was simply told, 'You don't need sleep to meditate,' so she carried on. But by the last day her sense of reality had become unhinged. 'I had all these sorts of strange thoughts about paranoia, and plots,' she tells me, on the phone from her home in Yorkshire. 'I felt very disconnected. But I think I still had an awareness at that point that it was a bit unusual, because at the end of the retreat there is a little tea party where everyone talks about their experience during the week, and I was going to say something about how I was feeling, and then I didn't because I thought it would sound peculiar.'

When she got home, things continued to deteriorate. 'We were having guests over,' she explains, 'and I was meant to pick them up from the station, but when I arrived to collect them I became convinced that they had bombs in their backpacks. It was the time of the IRA, so maybe that's what I was thinking – but I just turned around and went home.' Her husband soon realised something was wrong and persuaded her to go to the GP, who quickly diagnosed her as psychotic and manic. But despite medication her illness persisted. Over the course of the next three years Jane would spend several months as an in-patient at psychiatric hospitals, and was unable to work. Her symptoms were eventually only alleviated by electroconvulsive therapy.

She has since returned to meditation – but not in the Zen tradition. Instead, she runs a website called 'meditate in safety', which has links to scientific studies about the potential negative effects of meditation, and provides downloadable leaflets about the risks of sitting in silence. When we talk, she has just finished facilitating a retreat herself, as a 'well-being officer'. 'My hope is that teachers running retreats will take a more responsible attitude,' she says, 'and be aware that anyone could get into trouble. On our retreats we make an announcement at the start of weekend that if anyone is having difficulties they should come and see me, and we'll give what support we can. We give them permission to break the routine. It's difficult to break the silence, but we give them permission right from the start. If you don't feel well, you must talk with somebody.'

As I talk to her, it strikes me that there doesn't seem to me to be that much difference between Deva Mitra's experiences in Spain and Jane's sense of dissociation during the Zen retreat – and yet one is labelled mental illness and another is seen simply as an expected side effect of looking deeply into the nature of consciousness. The difference perhaps is that after the initial throes, Deva Mitra could control his symptoms, whereas Jane's life spiralled out of her control. Another crucial difference seems to be choice: Deva Mitra chose to break his silence. He asked for help. Just as Jane now advises novice meditators to do. The danger is when the silence can't be broken – like when

Jane thought her friends were carrying a bomb, and she lost all sense of reality.

The variety of experiences people have in silence seems at times overwhelming. But as I read, I learn there is a man who believes he can 'map' this territory, and make sense of what is happening to people like Jane or Anna, whose experiences run away with them in silence.

He is called Daniel Ingram, and claims he is an Arahat – someone who has reached enlightenment. His website carries a heavy disclaimer about getting in touch, urging you not to bother unless you have a question about meditation practice, or your own particular stage of enlightenment. He makes no secret of the fact that he is busy and is irked by intrusions on his time. By day he works as an emergency-room doctor, and by night he runs a community of Buddhists several thousand strong called the Dharma Overground. It was he who helped Anna to make sense of her experiences, while she was recovering from depression, by explaining to her that what was happening to her followed a predictable pattern and had been experienced by many other people.

I manage to speak to him over Skype late one evening, and he tells me that crossing over into 'dark night territory' doesn't always happen after months in silence; he knows of people in the Dharma Overground community who experienced this when driving their car, or during a massage. 'I know someone who was an actress and she was just doing this breath control workshop,' he says, 'and the next time she stepped on stage she had this explosion of consciousness – she wasn't on a retreat or anything.'

He says typically 'dark night' experiences will follow some-thing called the 'Arising and Passing Away', which he describes as a stage of human development that people may or may not undergo during their lives.[22] 'It is an attentional development stage akin to adolescence or puberty,' he tells me, 'when consciousness opens to deeper levels of perception.' And once that threshold has been crossed, the perception of the world shifts dramatically – and can lead to challenging experiences of dissociation, depression and fear. 'When it first happens, it is weird and disorientating,' he says, 'as these experiences begin to make what looked like a stable sense of self seem like a more transient, complicated, intricate, moving thing. That's what the Arising and Passing Away does; you see sensations arise and pass away – so you see the sensations that make up your sense of self arise and vanish, and that is a disconcerting thing for people who are used to their sense of self being continuous and stable.'

Once you have crossed this threshold, it can be terrifying; he tells me about people from the Dharma Overground who have crashed their cars on the way home from a yoga class, after suddenly crossing the 'Arising and Passing Away'. He knows people who became psychotic. Broken relationships are typical. Many people leave their jobs or find life just doesn't work in the same way. He describes these experiences as like pregnancy; with the right support and an understanding of what is happening, it can be a rich and rewarding experience, but if you don't know what is happening to your body it is petrifying[23] – a little bit like the girl buried in unconsecrated ground, scared to death of her periods. The crucial thing, Daniel says, is for people to talk about these experiences. In part this has been the role of the Dharma Overground – to allow people to talk about their experiences of meditation, including those that are difficult to articulate, and even taboo. He is, like Eve Ensler, evangelical about bringing the unsaid into plain sight. 'What's interesting,' he says, 'is that it's such a common phenomena. I mean, when you start talking about this stuff, people are like, "My God, this happened to me!" It happens to a lot of people, and yet somehow it's totally off the radar of modern medicine and psychology. I mean, you are starting to see trickles of it in the fringe edgy journals, but it has not reached the major journals like *The Lancet* or anything. It's a broadly reported human phenomena – and it's not on the radar screen yet.'

One of his interests is in 'mapping' these experiences to create a step-by-step guide to the path to enlightenment, so that people can make sense of what is happening to them, and compare and contrast their own experiences. As a result, he collects the experiences of meditators like a magpie picking through a hoard. And without warning the conversation pivots towards me.

'So what about you, then? Have you ever experienced any intense meditation experiences?' he asks.

I can feel the blood in my face. I want to distance myself from this talk about thresholds of consciousness and experience maps. I'm not sure I believe in any of it. But I have to say something.

'Well, yes, actually,' I begin.

And then I am telling him, articulating something I have never told anybody before. The anonymity of the phone helps, and perhaps the late-evening darkness outside lends an intimacy to our conversation I had not expected.

'I first knew I was bisexual when I was meditating,' I say.

Even as I say it, it sounds absurd. I have never admitted this fact to anyone; or found the words to say that it was while meditating that I knew, beyond doubt, that I found women attractive. It was during a lunchtime meditation, when things with my friend were getting increasingly difficult. My mother and several friends had asked if we were an item. I knew I had to say something, but didn't quite know what.

It was not a particularly intense meditation session – twenty minutes with the promise of tea and a biscuit afterwards. My mind was floating idly through the stages of the practice, watching the invisible spaces where my breath ended and began, and suddenly there was a rush of energy. Reading back through old diary entries, I described it as a surge of energy in my legs, moving up through my chest – a sense of heat. And I knew. It was a strange sensation, viscerally knowing something that had always been there: the certain knowledge that I found women sexually attractive – no images, no story; just a deeply felt and embodied truth. I have never experienced anything like it. And I can't help but feel words don't do it justice.

I have shied away from this story. Breaking it down into words, it sounds absurd. Perhaps because I don't know anyone else this has happened to. I have nothing to compare it with. I suppose that's why The Vagina Monologues matter. Or why Daniel's maps of meditation are important, because they offer people stories they can relate to. There is something so human in needing to know you're not alone, and it's that that gives you the courage to speak. So that, perhaps, language can take you closer to your experiences – and not further from them.

And then there is the fear. The fear of sharing the deeply private; that in sharing it will become meaningless and be explained away into nothing. Like Mary Oppen refusing to write directly about the experience of giving birth, as it was too direct and primal for words. I am not saying meditation made me sexually attracted to women, all I know is that sitting in silence, something that had always been there suddenly became obvious. I couldn't stay on the pillow. I opened my eyes. The heat and energy were still there. My rational mind was already whirring with stories about how this made sense and what I had to do now. I knew it then, and I couldn't change it. I understand Anna's magic-eye analogy. I couldn't go back to just seeing the dots. It was the inciting incident for everything that followed.

A week later I told my family that I liked women. I remember sitting with my grandmother in her study, and not offering any room for doubt. I think that's what people found strange. I wasn't 'experimenting'; I knew with an absolute certainty. But I didn't let anyone see this piece of the puzzle. So they had an incomplete version of events, which never quite made sense. I held something back, needing to maintain some vestige of control. A final breath of silence.

And so I tell Daniel about the feeling in my legs and stomach and needing to get out of the room. And how, after that, I changed everything else in my life. I could not ignore it.

'Classic A and P!' he says. 'Heightened sexual feelings – often non-heterosexual feelings – are very common.'

I have always been ashamed of this experience, as I couldn't explain how the sure knowledge of being bisexual came from meditation. Language had failed me. It is strange listening to Daniel talk about this experience as akin to crossing a threshold of consciousness – he jokes that all the existentialist thinkers would have crossed the A and P – as to hold contradictory thoughts in your head you had to have walked this territory. I'm not sure I buy into the idea that this rush of energy was a form of enlightenment. But that first telling prompted others, as words so often do. Stories beget stories. Words beget words. Unknotting the power of the experience.

PART FIVE

LAST WORD

THAT THIS IS I, NOT MINE

WHEN I WENT BACK TO Scotland on silent retreat, I said I was going to investigate silence. But I also went on retreat as I was getting married, and I wanted to understand – or at least be aware of – the experience of being alone, before this greatest change in my life. Marriage reforms the self into a new unit. It is the event at the end of Shakespeare's comedies and the start of the tragedies: a pivot on which the plot turns. I wanted the stillness before the spin.

It seemed right to spend time in silence before getting married. I could think of few other occasions where language occupies such a privileged position. Making the marriage vows is one of the rare moments when language is not merely descriptive – it changes things in the world. The words themselves are an object – participating in the world of objects; not just a cipher between self and world.

I wanted to see where I was before that. A return to the pre-linguistic swamp before putting my faith in the spoken vows: I do.

A lot of the retreat focused on the cultivation of *metta*, which is roughly translated from the Pali as 'loving kindness'. We would sit in silence, wishing that both ourselves and all living beings could be happy and well. One of the Buddhists I spoke to told me this state promoted a feeling of opening up, and that it was through this experience of well-wishing that we glimpse non-duality – that is, when feeling generous and open, we have a sense of the self unfolding into the other.

During one of these meditations we were asked to visualise our hearts as a cave. I flinched at the idea of visualisation, as I had never done it before. But they gave examples to help guide us: the cave might be a cavern in the high hewn rock, they said, or a safe hermitage, or an *Arabian Nights* fantasy of hidden treasure. My mind began to wander. I was honestly unsure how to equate my heart with a cave. Then suddenly I had a strong sense of the sea – of a hollow in the sandstone cliffs of the North Devon coast. I felt the wet winter sand underfoot, the cement-like footprints and hair whipped into my mouth by the wind. I could see my brother and I jumping from the sand dunes as children under a grey December sky. I was at my grandmother's flat, which we had stayed in every half-term and school holiday as children. And there were smells, before all else, like the old sea air in the garage, where the walls were damp with salt. I remembered going rock-pooling, and scraping at the weed underwater, before pushing jelly-like shrimps into our plastic buckets; smashing mussels on the rocks to fish for crabs; and walking out along the disused sewage pipe with our grisly harvest; lowering our nets into the dark water and pulling up crabs as big as a fist, fighting over each other to reach the bait. The other children gathering around to look. And inside my grandmother's flat, the thick white rug by the gas fire where the red bulbs of the electric fireplace turned. Watching the same three or four videos where the film skipped and scratched, rendered senseless by the repetition.

It was strange that my mind had taken me there. A place of profound safety – before senior school, and the boot room and silence. Before all of this. When asked to visualise the heart, that is where I went – back to my family, to the space before the silence.

I had met my fiancée one year after my first retreat. At first I didn't tell her how recently I had come out. I made up another story. Gay marriage had just been legalised and it was a moment of bright possibility, my friends said. Being bisexual shouldn't be such a big deal. On our second date, my girlfriend asked what I thought about marriage equality. During a walk through frost-bitten Greenwich she told me that she felt 'gay' was a redundant qualifier – it was like saying we were having 'gay' lunch. It was just lunch. And marriage was just marriage. At the time I said I didn't know what I thought. I couldn't imagine how the word could be elastic enough to include two women being married. I think I said something clever about the word being loaded with heteronormative garbage and chained to patriarchal control. But to be honest, when we went on our first date I really didn't know what sex was like between two women – let alone marriage. Again, the words were not plastic enough to match the fast-evolving reality.

During our first conversation about gay marriage, on our second date, I remember our fingers – interlaced yet barely touching. Slurred and hazy with wine, we sat opposite each other, the tips of our fingers just grazing – gesturing at the promise of physical intimacy. We couldn't and didn't kiss in public. She had grown up as a lesbian in the nineties, when public displays of affection were less common, and the habit ran deep. She had known people to shout abuse in the street. She wanted me to be sure. So she made me kiss her first. Despite my bravado, she sensed that none of it was real. She needed me to reach into it. To say yes.

So we had a date in her one-bedroom not-quite flat. She had travelled across London to buy a second chair, as she only had one. There was a peculiarly Scandinavian economy to her kitchen: there was one sharp knife, a small pan and a big pan. One of everything, a little life. I fried onions for ragu, and drank so much wine I could barely speak straight. I tried to explain that I had only come out a few months earlier. That although I had been on dates – so many dates – and had joined endless 'Meetup' groups to try and meet other gay, queer, bi-curious women, nothing had happened. I often left the groups with a feeling that I might as well have tried to meet other tall women; sexuality seemed an utterly arbitrary indicator that we would have anything in common.

We kissed at the last possible moment that evening. I remember I could encircle her waist with my arms. And I cried with relief on the night bus through Elephant and Castle. Because I had been right.

Of course, the years that followed were marked by our share of flowers and flint; and at one stage we sat opposite each other in a rowing boat, while I told her I wanted to break up. I didn't really – I just wanted to make peace with being with women. The loss of the imagined future took a long time to adapt to, and part of that was because I was raised on stories of handsome princes and brave knights. The imagined shape of my future was peopled with men, and in some ways the hardest thing was imagining that life could look different.

We got engaged in the rain in Seville two years after the argument in the rowing boat. Neither of us had imagined that we would get married. The bouffant white blancmange was too much, and until so recently marriage had been a legal impossibility. But it felt important somehow to say yes. The world was changing. She was nursing her mother through the final stages of cancer and the good things seemed gossamer-precarious.

We registered the engagement in Peckham three months later. I had not known that the names of everyone who registers to be married would be flashed up on the TV screen in the registry office. As we waited our turn, we watched the names roll past – laughing and guessing how they might have met. Almost but not all the names were male and female pairings. We never saw our names on the screen. But it felt good that they were there – for tomorrow's couples to see. In some ways it felt like an end to the uncertainty; to the slow curl of coming out, to the not-knowing. It signalled an end to this part of the story – to see our names, and the promise of marriage, there in black and white.

It was in the days after registering the engagement that I chose the George Oppen poem to read at the wedding. I loved the tale of the Oppens' impetuous romance, and was happy to tether our story to theirs. I imagined George in the car with Mary, driving through France or sailing into New York. The wind and salt and hopes of a generation – before the rise of fascism and the dark clouds of war.

When George and Mary got married, they were on the run from George's parents. Despite the endless dinner parties and chandeliers, they felt suffocated by his parents' wealth, and moved away to start their own lives. As Mary remembers, 'A girl we met gave me her purple velvet dress. Her boyfriend gave us a pint of gin . . . we bought a ten cent ring and went to the ugly red courthouse that still stands in Dallas.'[1] And then they were 'a mated pair' – as Mary says, the rest 'inevitable'. I have always loved the irreverence of their wedding: in ill-fitting, hastily borrowed clothes with a ten-cent ring; the ceremony strangely irrelevant. It was the life ahead that mattered.

The poem I chose seemed to capture their sense of optimism for the future. As I read it, I imagined them that first night, when George sneaked into Mary's college dorm and they drove away and talked until morning, an intimation of all that could be it begins.

That this is I,
Not mine, which wakes
To where the present
Sun pours in the present, to the air perhaps
Of love and of
Conviction.[2]

What I had not realised is how episodic my memory of the day would be. It is piecemeal in my mind: I remember buying flowers in the morning – walking to the florist and telling her I was getting married in an hour. Delighting in the words, and sense of expectation. Then holding the flowers in a plastic bag so the water didn't leak.

The rest of the day is glimpses. There is a string caught in my dress, being pulled straight outside the registry office. My girlfriend running outside to ask her sister what her father's profession had been in English. The clerk fiddling with his fountain pen. He looked like a schoolboy in his blazer.

I had intended to end this story with choosing language; saying 'I do'. A final and defiant emergence from the uncertainty of silence.

But the fact is, I can't actually remember what we said. We had not written our own vows and instead spoke the ones they give you at the registry office – on a laminated piece of paper passed from hand to hand. We wanted to participate in a ritual bigger than our own made-up promises. So the words were demotic. Spoken, not written. Not premeditated. And somehow that was important. Like the words spoken in a Quaker meeting, they arose from and disappeared back into, the silence, like pebbles in a pool.

The moments I remember are more physical: the registrar asking us to hold hands. I didn't know we would be told to do that. I remember taking my new wife's hands and being transported straight back to that second date. The fingertips, the wine – the first physical intimation that I had been right, and that all the telling and re-telling had been worth it.

And I remember trying out the word 'wife' in a café afterwards, feeling its weight on my tongue as we ate poached eggs. Then coming home, peeling off our tights and taking the dog out in the park. An ending of sorts. Or a beginning.

THE FACES OF STRANGERS

GEORGE OPPEN'S STORY ALSO ENDED in the things that could not be said. He developed Alzheimer's and gradually lost the ability to speak. The world became a terrifying place. You can see it in his later letters, as he turns down appointments, unsure if he will even be able to get there. When invited to speak at an event by Paul Auster in 1980, he wrote:

> Very tempting – a pleasant prospect to see you again, and to talk. What worries me is the question of whether or not I can say anything that I have not already said – And my own condition at this moment which is something alas, very like senility . . . It is not that I fear being less than brilliant: I find that my only recourse is to admit to myself and to others that on familiar streets I cannot find my way home.[3]

Although he was not diagnosed with the disease until the 1980s, the tell-tale signs salt his correspondence, for in one letter written in 1976 he admitted that 'little can be expected from my memory since I become confused so easily even in the narrative present'.[4] And even as early as 1974 he confessed to another correspondent that he was increasingly unable to recognise the faces of people he knew well. He and Mary were spending the summer sailing in Maine, and although 'We talk to people on this island – people we've seen every summer for ten years', Mary has to 'whisper their names to me as they approach and I forget them again before I can say hello. It's getting strange, it's becoming strange.'[5] As the correspondence continues, he tracks the deterioration of the condition, writing, 'Senility: no other word for it. I cannot remember what happened yesterday . . . 67: a little early for such things – I cannot do simple arithmetic. I misread clocks . . . Been talking to a doctor: he begins with no coffee, no tea, no alcohol, and of course no tobacco, but I don't find that possible – I see myself walking about supported by Mary's elbow – pretty soon (Or is Mary's elbow a stimulant and therefore forbidden?)'[6]

In her Preface to the last few letters Oppen wrote, his biographer Rachel Blau DuPlessis says that during these years of confusion the Oppens wrote letters to each other to try and work out what was happening and what they should do. They needed the words to hang onto.

There is something so moving about these lifelong partners – who would habitually finish each other's sentences – having to write letters to each other in order to communicate. And fittingly, perhaps, they are not published.[7] This final private correspondence was better left unsaid.

The tragedy is that the disease seemed to take Oppen further away from the world he loved so much. Faces were unknowable, familiar streets strange. This was a new silence. Not the space between the little words that allowed a deeper communion with the world – but one of fear and, ultimately, death.[8]

And so Oppen has brought me full circle – to the lonely and isolated silence that somehow distorts identity; a man who cannot find his way home, and a little girl standing by the cloaks in the boot room.

*

Looking back at my time writing about silence in the quiet of the library, where you exist in symbiosis with the people around you, I am reminded of something my father said after the Paddington rail crash. He had commuted along the same line for decades and told me he missed the faces of the people he had come to recognise during the commute, after they perished. They were known to him somehow. The other people in the library were like that to me. We worked alongside each other all day, but never spoke. I didn't know who they were, but they were part of the shape of my life – separated by silence. And all those years ago, in the boot room, it was silence that kept me both from the self I remembered as a child, and also from other people. But I have learnt that silence is more complicated. It can be dehumanising, but it can also help to build communities, whether within a convent or on retreat, as without language we have less to separate us from each other. In the process of writing I have come to value silence, to sink down into it each morning at my desk. It feels clarifying – like the slow settlement of silt on a river bed, somehow filtering my thoughts.

When Oppen looked back over his own extended silence, he said that there were simply 'some things [he] had to live through, some things [he] had to think [his] way through, some things [he] had to try out' before he could write again, so that 'in brief, it just took twenty-five years to write the next poem'.[9] And infuriating as this answer is, in many ways I understand Oppen's logic, and the idea that words are of their time. They can't be written any earlier. I certainly know I could not have written this before. For I feel as though I am writing from the other side – looking back through the porthole glass, to borrow one of Oppen's favourite images – at everything that has happened. Seeing the turbulence from a place of safety.

I can see now that as a child I stopped talking because of shame – because I was told not to – and I knew from a very young age that the details of your private life should remain behind closed doors. And to be honest, I have struggled with that throughout the writing of this book, exploring what should and should not remain unsaid. It has been difficult bringing these aspects of my life into the air, making them real; writing about events which I feel are not truly my own, but the stories of the unnamed friends and exes and, above all, of my family. In the process of writing this I have come to understand more than ever the appeal of silence – you can't get it wrong, or distort someone else's story, if you refuse to say anything. And as I approach the end of this journey, I am not sure if the act of telling stories and articulating events makes things any more real – or if in the process of telling we inevitably distort. I suspect the act of recalling memories changes them, and then telling bends them further out of shape, so that you are left with something akin to the face we make when we know we are looking in a mirror. Life as it is lived is closer to the unexpected glance in the swimming-pool changing room, the spare flesh, the confusion and the feeling of 'how did that happen?'

And yet, I must hold onto the fact that there is a value in telling – in bearing witness as a journalist, and also telling in the unfettered confidentiality of Samaritans. It can be transformative, as Eve Ensler found out when encouraging women to name the taboo and the unspeakable, and as countless callers have learnt when faced with the benevolent darkness on the end of the telephone. Speaking about your experiences can help bring order to chaos, as it did for the woman in Nepal, whose world had literally fallen apart. Despite the inevitable distortion of telling, there is still a value in trying to explain what has happened.

So this is where this particular story – of emergence from silence into spoken certainty – ends: in a registry office on the Peckham Road on the last warm day of summer. And with Oppen, the poet of the gaps, the glances, the things unsaid. It feels like an ending – an act of standing up and saying this is who I am. I never did stand on stage and say the word 'vagina' – in a funny way, this may be the closest I will ever get.

I can't tell you if silence is any better than talking – the truth is, I don't think they can be separated that easily. They inevitably overlap, and bleed into each other. I have learned that part of telling is keeping secrets – about the unnamed exes, the unmentioned locations. I was frequently floored by the way, as I spoke to people, they would tell me unrepeatable things: ending an interview with the utterly unexpected revelation that they had tried to kill themselves, or had been blackmailed. Some comments were said off the record, and for others I had to decide to leave them out – with the understanding that life is a quilt of secrets. And it's not up to us to unpick it, or the whole thing falls apart. The trust of telling – of writing or speaking stories – is keeping other people's secrets. I know that now. There are so many things I have left out. Some omissions prey on my mind. I wish I had said earlier how my family's understanding of words developed and expanded: how they changed their view of what makes a family or a marriage. And how grateful I am for that expansion, for the plasticity of their thinking – and for their love: the handful of baby teeth, saved for a lifetime. I can only hope they know.

Writing is always sifting through what can and cannot be said: the off-the-record comments, the edges of other people's stories, the locked archives. So that each new act of telling can only ever gesture towards everything that has not been said. Or, as Oppen would say:

> say as much as I dare, as much as I can
> sustain I don't know how to say it
>
> I say all that I can[10]

NOTES

PART ONE: FEAR

1 'George Oppen interviewed by L. S. Dembo, Madison, Wisconsin, April 25, 1968', *Speaking with George Oppen: Interviews with the Poet and Mary Oppen, 1968–1987*, edited by Richard Swigg (Jefferson, NC, and London: McFarland and Company, 2012), p. 10.

2 'Objectivist' in 'Glossary of Poetic Terms', see Poetry Foundation website: www.poetryfoundation.org; accessed 10 May 2018.

3 'Psalm', George Oppen, *New Collected Poems* (New York: New Directions, 2002; Manchester: Carcanet Press, 2003), p. 99.

4 'George Oppen interviewed by L. S. Dembo, Madison, Wisconsin, April 25, 1968', *Speaking with George Oppen*, p. 11.

5 Oppen, 'Of Being Numerous', *New Collected Poems*, p. 166.

6 Oppen, 'Of Being Numerous', *New Collected Poems*, p. 171.

7 Ezra Pound, 'Preface to *Discrete Series*' (1934), George Oppen, *New Collected Poems* (New York: New Directions, 2002; Manchester: Carcanet Press, 2003), p. 4.

8 Oppen, from *Discrete Series* in *New Collected Poems*, p. 13.

9 Oppen, from *Discrete Series* in *New Collected Poems*, p. 29.

10 Oppen, from *Discrete Series* in *New Collected Poems*, p. 7.

11 Oppen, from *Discrete Series* in *New Collected Poems*, p. 9.

12 *The Selected Letters of George Oppen*, edited by Rachel Blau DuPlessis (Durham, NC, and London: Duke University Press, 1990).

13 DuPlessis, 'Introduction', *The Selected Letters of George Oppen*, pp. vii–xx.

14 For details of these early travels, and the Oppens' time in France, see Mary Oppen, *Meaning a Life, an Autobiography* (Boston, MA: Black Sparrow Press, 1978), pp. 117–41.

15 'I think it was fifteen million families that were faced with the threat of imminent starvation. It wasn't a business you simply read about in the newspaper. You stepped out of your door and found men who had nothing to eat.' 'George Oppen interviewed by L. S. Dembo, Madison, Wisconsin, April 25, 1968', *Speaking with George Oppen*, p. 20.

16 Peter Nicholls, *George Oppen and the Fate of Modernism* (Oxford: Oxford University Press, 2007), p. 17.

17 George Oppen, 'The Mind's Own Place', *Selected Poems* (New York: New Directions, 1962), see www.poetryfoundation.org/articles/69407/the-minds-own-place; accessed May 2018.

18 The phrase 'a spectre in every street' appears in 'Blood from a stone,' in Oppen, *New Collected Poems*, p. 52.

19 Oppen, 'Of Being Numerous', *New Collected Poems*, p. 163.

20 Oppen, 'Semantic', in 'Selected Unpublished Poems', *New Collected Poems*, p. 336.

21 The image *Christmas in Manhattan, 1931* can be viewed at 'The Great Depression and New Deal' under the subheading 'Breadlines'. See <https://infograph.venngage.com/p/190738/the-great-depression-and-new-deal>

22 George Oppen, '"Meaning Is to Be Here": A Selection from the Daybook', *Conjunctions:10* (Spring 1987), edited by Bradford Morrow, p. 197.

23 Mary Oppen, *Meaning a Life*, p. 151.

24 'The political crisis of unemployment and poverty galvanised them. They worked as organisers for a social change which was democratic socialist and populist in its ultimate contours, but also committed to the class analysis of Marxism'. Rachel Blau DuPlessis, 'Introduction', *The Selected Letters of George Oppen*, p. 9.

25 'George Oppen interviewed by L. S. Dembo' in *Speaking with George Oppen*, p. 21.

26 DuPlessis, 'Introduction', *The Selected Letters of George Oppen*, p. 14.

27 'Because of his resistance to the instrumental use of artists within the party Oppen concealed his vocation and soon stopped writing.' DuPlessis, 'Introduction', *The Selected Letters of George Oppen*, p. 13.

28 'George Oppen interviewed by L. S. Dembo, Madison, Wisconsin, April 25, 1968', *Speaking with George Oppen*, p. 20.

29 Burton Hatlen and Tom Mandel, 'Poetry and Politics: A conversation with George and Mary Oppen', *George Oppen, Man and Poet*, edited by Burton Hatlen (University of Maine: National Poetry Foundation, 1981), p. 25.

30 *The Selected Letters of George Oppen*, edited by Rachel Blau DuPlessis, p. 207.

31 'From the moment I stepped into [June's] house I saw something of the luxury into which George was born and from which he tried to escape.' This observation was made by Michael Davidson in 'Distant Life', *The Oppens Remembered: Poetry, Politics, and Friendship*, edited by Rachel Blau DuPlessis (Albuquerque: University of New Mexico Press, 2015), p. 107.

32 'They lived in a marble palace . . . to my childish eyes a horrible long echoing, vast non-home. It was like going to a bank or maybe a hotel.' This observation was made by Linda Oppen, recalling

visiting her paternal grandparents (George's parents) in San Francisco. See 'Turquoise', *The Oppens Remembered*, p. 229.

33 'Notes from Memoirs and Conversations of Julian Zimet', *The Oppens Remembered*, p. 7.

34 'Conversation with Mary Oppen', *The Iowa Review*, Vol. 8: Issue 3 (Fall 1988), p. 22.

35 For details of the 'quiet-turned' children, see David Looff, *Appalachia's Children: The Challenge of Mental Health* (Lexington, KY: University of Kentucky Press, 1971).

36 The official NHS guidance also notes that '[SM] is more common in girls and children of ethnic minority populations, or in those who have recently migrated from their country of birth.' NHS, 'Selective Mutism', August 2014; see www.nhs.uk/conditions/selective-mutism; accessed August 2016. The one in 150 figure falls to around one in 1000 adolescents, and according to some research (see Carl Sutton, 'An Experiential Introduction to Selective Mutism', *Selected Mutism in Our Own Words, Experiences in Childhood and Adulthood*, edited by Carl Sutton and Cheryl Forrester (London: Jessica Kingsley Publishers, 2015) SM affects up to one in 2,400 young adults.

37 In 'Introducing Selective Mutism and an Overview of Approaches', in Benita Rae Smith and Alice Sluckin (eds), *Tackling Selective Mutism* (London: Jessica Kingsley Publishers, 2015), p. 18, Alice Sluckin, the founder of SMIRA, notes that SM is often initially misdiagnosed as 'separation anxiety' in very young children and that a child with SM may have 'difficulty making eye contact' at school and can therefore 'appear withdrawn and defensive'. And in Carl Sutton and Cheryl Forrester, *Selective Mutism in Our Own Words* (London: Jessica Kingsley Publishers, 2015), p. 16, Carl Sutton, himself a former SM sufferer, observes that SM is 'most frequently noted in the school environment'.

38 For example, Sheila A. Spasaro and Charles E. Schaefer's SM treatment manual, which was published as late as 1999 – several years after SM had been classified as an anxiety disorder by the World Health Organization – is tellingly titled *Refusal to Speak: Treatment of Selective Mutism in Children*.

39 See *A Clinical Lesson at the Salpêtrière* by Pierre Aristide André Brouillet, 1887. See <https://en.wikipedia.org/wiki/A_Clinical_Lesson_at_the_Salp%C3%AAtri%C3%A8re>

40 This account of hysteria and the Salpêtrière hospital is based on Asti Hustvedt's fascinating book *Medical Muses: Hysteria in Nineteenth Century Paris* (New York: W. W. Norton & Co.; London: Bloomsbury, 2011).

41 Hustvedt, *Medical Muses*, p. 53.

42 Hustvedt, *Medical Muses*, p. 26.

43 'Charcot did nothing less than pave the way for psychoanalysis', Hustvedt, *Medical Muses*, p. 62.

44 This argument is outlined by Rachel Bowlby in her Introduction to Sigmund Freud and Josef Breuer's *Studies in Hysteria*, translated by Nicola Luckhurst (London: Penguin, 2004).

45 The details of this story are based on the account given by Tony Cline in 'Selective Mutism in Children: Changing Perspective Over Half a Century', in Smith and Sluckin (eds), *Tackling Selective Mutism*, pp. 34–51.

46 In so doing he was drawing on the ideas of German neurologist Adolf Kussmaul, who had first described the condition as '*Aphasia Voluntaria*', the Latin term meaning 'voluntary lack of speech', in 1877. See Smith and Sluckin (eds), *Tackling Selective Mutism*, p. 35. (Kussmaul also identified dyslexia as 'word blindness' at about the same time.)

47 The name 'Selective Mutism' was 'decisively adopted by the American Psychiatric Association in 1994' (see Cline, 'Selective

Mutism in Children: Changing Perspective Over Half a Century', Smith and Sluckin (eds), *Tackling Selective Mutism*, pp. 35–6). However, Cline also points out that some therapists in the US had been calling the condition 'selective mutism' since the mid 1970s (p. 34) 'with no published explanation', and that a team in New York state referred to it as 'speech phobia' as early as 1971.

48 See, for example, Maggie Johnson's books (with Alison Wintgens), *Can I tell you about Selective Mutism* (London: Jessica Kingsley Publishers, 2012) and *The Selective Mutism Resource Manual* (Abingdon: Routledge, 2001).

49 For more on the functioning of the amygdala, see Bruno Dubuc, 'The Amygdala and Its Allies' and 'Two Pathways of Fear'; at <thebrain.mcgill.ca/flash/a/a_04/a_04_cr/a_04_cr_peu/a_04_cr_peu. html>

50 Norman MacCaig, 'Aunt Julia', *The Many Days: Selected Poems of Norman MacCaig* (Edinburgh: Polygon, 2010).

51 This story is told in Mary Oppen's biography, *Meaning a Life*, p. 202.

52 Rachel Blau DuPlessis, 'Introduction' to *The Selected Letters of George Oppen*, pp. 15–17.

53 Linda Oppen, 'Turquoise', *The Oppens Remembered*, p. 238.

54 For more on the Oppens' time in Mexico, see Nicholls, *George Oppen and the Fate of Modernism*, p. 25.

55 Mary Oppen, *Meaning a Life*, pp. 194–5.

56 Mary Oppen, *Meaning a Life*, p. 197.

57 Mary Oppen, *Meaning a Life*, pp. 198–9.

58 Linda Oppen, 'Turquoise', *The Oppens Remembered*, p. 239.

59 Mary Oppen, *Meaning a Life*, p. 200.

60 This methodology is described in Stephen Cope's Introduction to Oppen's *Selected Prose, Daybooks, and Papers* (Oakland, CA: University of California Press, 2007), pp. 14–17.

61 George Oppen, 'The Mind's Own Place', *Selected Poems*.

62 'George Oppen interviewed by L. S. Dembo', *Speaking with George Oppen*, p. 11.

63 For a more thorough account of how SM can affect adults, I would recommend Carl Sutton and Cheryl Forrester's book, *Selective Mutism in Our Own Words*, which gathers the testimony of many adult SM sufferers, including Carl himself.

64 Marjorie Wallace, *The Silent Twins* (London: Vintage, 1998), p. 17.

65 Wallace, *The Silent Twins*, p. 46.

66 The names of all children and their families have been changed to protect their identities.

67 For Jon's first-hand account of his recovery from SM, see Jonathan Kohlmeier, *Learning to Play the Game: My Journey Through Silence* (Morrisville, NC: Lulu Publishing Services, 2016).

PART TWO: SEX

1 George Oppen, '"Meaning Is to Be Here": A Selection from the Daybook', *Conjunctions:10* (Spring 1987), edited by Bradford Morrow, p. 198.

2 Mary Oppen, *Meaning a Life, an Autobiography* (Boston, MA: Black Sparrow Press, 1978), p. 61.

3 Mary Oppen, *Meaning a Life*, p. 62.

4 George Oppen, 'The Forms of Love', *New Collected Poems* (New York: New Directions, 2002; Manchester: Carcanet Press, 2003), p. 106.

5 Mary Oppen, *Meaning a Life*, p. 63. The other details of this meeting are all drawn from Mary's account in her autobiography.

6 Burton Hatlen, 'Introduction', *George Oppen, Man and Poet*, edited by Burton Hatlen (University of Maine: National Poetry Foundation, 1981), p. 5.

7   Mary Oppen, *Meaning a Life*, p. 76.

8   Eve Ensler, 'Hair', *The Vagina Monologues, 20th Anniversary Edition* (London: Virago Press, 2018), p. 8.

9   Ensler, *The Vagina Monologues*, p. 9.

10 Laura Barnett, Interview with Eve Ensler, 'How We Made: The *Vagina Monologues*', *The Guardian*, 4 February 2013.

11 Eve Ensler, 'Introduction to the 20th Anniversary Edition', *The Vagina Monologues*, p. xi.

12 James Langton, 'Stars come out for V-Day', *Daily Telegraph*, 14 February 1998.

13 'Hoohaa in US over Monologues play', BBC News website, 9 February 2007.

14 Eve Ensler, *Insecure at Last: Losing It in Our Security-obsessed World*, (New York: Villard Books, 2006), p. xvi.

15 Ensler, *Insecure at Last*, p. xvi.

16 George Oppen, '"Meaning Is to Be Here": A Selection from the Daybook', p. 193.

17 George Oppen, '"Meaning Is to Be Here": A Selection from the Daybook', p. 193.

18 George Oppen, '"Meaning Is to Be Here": A Selection from the Daybook', p. 195.

19 George Oppen, '"Meaning Is to Be Here": A Selection from the Daybook', p. 193.

20 George Oppen, 'Route', *New Collected Poems*, p. 193.

21 George Oppen, 'Of Being Numerous', *New Collected Poems*, p. 182.

22 Susan Celia Swan and Purva Panday Cullman, 'Say It, Stage It, V-Day at Twenty', *The Vagina Monologues, 20th Anniversary Edition*, p. 176.

23 Swan and Cullman, 'Say It, Stage It, V-Day at Twenty', p. 179.

24 'Eve Ensler: The Power of Story' podcast, Sydney Opera House,

12 December 2017. See <https://www.sydneyoperahouse.com/backstage/podcasts/its-a-long-story/eve-ensler.html>; accessed January 2018.

25 George Oppen, 'Route', *New Collected Poems*, p. 193.

26 The details of Sophie Andrews' life are drawn from her book *Scarred* (London: Hodder & Stoughton, 2007).

27 Sophie Andrews, 'The Interview', BBC World Service, 7 March 2010. See <https://www.bbc.co.uk/programmes/p006g30n>; accessed January 2018.

28 The details of this story are drawn from the TV documentary *Chad Varah: The Good Samaritan* (August 1992).

29 Chad Varah, *Before I Die Again* (London: Constable, 1992).

30 Chad Varah interviewed by Niamh Dillon for the *National Life Stories: Pioneers in Charity and Social Welfare* series, audio recordings, 2004-12-09 and 2005-01-05. Accessed at British Library Sound Archive.

31 For an excellent account of some of the taboos around menstruation in Nepal, see Rose George, 'Blood Speaks', in *Mosaic*, 11 March 2014. See <https://mosaicscience.com/story/menstrual-taboo-periods-shame-women/>

32 Chad Varah, *Before I Die Again*, p. 83.

33 Chad Varah, *Before I Die Again*, p. 112.

34 'Sex and the Citizen', *Picture Post*, 15 September 1951: *Picture Post* Historical Archive; accessed 2 August 2018.

35 *Chad Varah: The Good Samaritan* (August 1992).

36 *Chad Varah: The Good Samaritan* (August 1992).

37 'A Parson Puts His Case', *Picture Post*, 10 November 1951: *Picture Post* Historical Archive; accessed 2 August 2018.

38 Chad Varah, *Before I Die Again*, p. 149.

39 Chad Varah, *Before I Die Again*, p. 150.

40 Chad Varah, *Before I Die Again*, p. 151.

41 Chad Varah, *Before I Die Again*, p. 153.

42 Chad Varah, *Before I Die Again*, p. 158.

43 This account of the formation of Samaritans is drawn from both the documentary *Chad Varah: The Good Samaritan* (August1992), and Chad's autobiography, *Before I Die Again*.

44 David G. Kibble, *The Samaritans*, Charities Series (Oxford: Pergamon Press, 1983), p. 11. Kibble explains that in 1964 there were 5,566 suicides in England and Wales, and by 1973 this had dropped to 3,821.

45 Michael Davidson, 'Introduction', George Oppen, *New Collected Poems* (New York: New Directions, 2002; Manchester: Carcanet Press, 2003), p. xxviii.

46 For further details of Frank Lake's work, Alan recommended F. J. Roberts, 'Clinical Theology: An Assessment', *Theological Students Fellowship (TSF) Bulletin*, Vol. 64 (Autumn 1972), pp. 21–5.

47 Mary Oppen, *Meaning a Life*, p. 167.

48 Mary Oppen, *Meaning a Life*, p. 167.

49 *The Selected Letters of George Oppen*, edited by Rachel Blau DuPlessis (Durham, NC, and London: Duke University Press, 1990), p. 35.

50 Mary Oppen, *Meaning a Life*, p. 98.

51 George Oppen, '"Meaning Is to Be Here": A Selection from the Daybook', p. 198.

52 Rachel Blau DuPlessis, 'Introduction', *The Selected Letters of George Oppen*, p. 11.

53 *The Selected Letters of George Oppen*, p. 353.

54 *The Selected Letters of George Oppen*, p. 35.

55 *Chad Varah: The Good Samaritan* (August 1992).

56 *Chad Varah: The Good Samaritan* (August 1992).

57 'Suicide Leading Cause of Death in Men aged 20–49 in England & Wales', Campaign Against Living Miserably (CALM), 18

February 2014. See <https://www.thecalmzone.net/2014/02/onssu-icidereport/ >; accessed January 2018.

58 Swan and Cullman, 'Say It, Stage It, V-Day at Twenty', p 186. 'The Democratic Republic of Congo has since 1996 endured the deadliest war since World War II. The conflict – a proxy war for Congo's vast natural resources has directed rampant violence . . . towards women. Advocates on the ground estimate that more than half a million women and girls have been raped since the conflict began', p. 187.

59 Eve Ensler, *In the Body of the World* (London: Virago Press, 2013), p. 16.

60 'Eve Ensler: The Power of Story' podcast.

61 Dr Mukwege was awarded the Nobel Peace Prize for his work in Congo in October 2018.

62 Eve Ensler, *In the Body of the World*, p. 16.

63 For more on City of Joy, see <http://drc.vday.org/about-city-of-joy>

64 'Eve Ensler: The Power of Story' podcast.

PART THREE: DEATH

1 For further information on the delays in government aid, see, for example, 'Nepal: Two years on, the government continues to fail marginalised earthquake survivors', *Amnesty International*, 25 April 2017. See <https://www.amnesty.org/en/latest/news/2017/04/nepal-two-years-on-the-government-continues-to-fail-marginalised-earth-quake-survivors/> or Jennifer Rigby, 'Nepal earthquake anniversary: one year on, not one home rebuilt by government', *Daily Telegraph*, 25 April 2016. See <https://www.telegraph.co.uk/news/2016/04/25/nepal-earthquake-anniversary-one-year-on-not-one-home-rebuilt-by/>

2 See, for example, C. Karki, 'Suicide: Leading Cause of Death among Women in Nepal', *Kathmandu University Medical Journal*,

Vol. 9: 3, Issue 35 (July–September 2011), pp. 157–8. The true level of suicide in Nepal is disputed, due to a lack of conclusive data, but according to a 2009 government survey, quoted in a WHO report: 'suicide (16%) rather than maternal-related issues (12%) was the single leading cause of death among more than 86,000 women of reproductive age in eight districts and of different ethnicities and levels of development', in K. Marahatta et al., 'Suicide burden and prevention in Nepal: the need for a national strategy', *WHO South East Asia Journal of Public Health*, 6:1 (April 2017), p. 46.

3   This story is recounted in 'Depression too is a thing with feathers' at www.andrewsolomon.com (January 2008); accessed March 2017.

4   The historian was Professor Edgar Jones and his arguments are explained in his excellent book (with Simon Wessely): *Shell Shock and PTSD: Military Psychiatry from 1900 to the Gulf War* (New York and Hove, Sussex: Psychology Press, 2005). For further information on shell shock, and the relationship between warfare and psychiatry, see also Ben Shephard's *A War of Nerves: Soldiers and Psychiatrists 1914–1994* (London: Jonathan Cape, 2000).

5   Percy Meek became a cause célèbre, and his case history is recorded by William McDougall in *An Outline of Abnormal Psychology* (London: Methuen & Co., 1926), pp. 289–92. He was also filmed by Arthur Hurst and appears in the groundbreaking film about the treatment of shell shock, *War Neuroses* (1917). Although, as Edgar Jones points out, some of the 'before' scenes showing soldiers unable to walk or talk may have been shot after the event. For more details, see Edgar Jones, 'War Neuroses and Arthur Hurst: a pioneering medical film about the treatment of psychiatric battle casualties', *Journal of the History of Medicine and Allied Sciences*, 67:3 (May 2011), pp. 345–73.

6   Sigmund Freud and Josef Breuer, *Studies in Hysteria*, translated by Nicola Luckhurst (London: Penguin, 2004). p. 34.

7   Freud and Breuer, *Studies in Hysteria*, p. 10.

8   C. S. Myers, 'A contribution to the study of shell shock', *The Lancet*, 13 February 1915, p. 316. See <http://jmvh.org/wp-content/uploads/2012/12/A-Contribution-to-the-Study-of-Shellshock.pdf>

9   Myers is cited by Edgar Jones and Simon Wessely, 'Battle for the Mind: World War 1 and the birth of military psychiatry', *The Lancet*, 8 November 2014, p. 1709. See <https://www.kcl.ac.uk/kcmhr/publications/assetfiles/2014/Jones2014e.pdf>

10 All these recollections are from Linda Oppen, 'Turquoise', *The Oppens Remembered: Poetry, Politics, and Friendship*, edited by Rachel Blau DuPlessis (Albuquerque: University of New Mexico Press, 2015), p. 225.

11 *The Selected Letters of George Oppen*, edited by Rachel Blau DuPlessis (Durham, NC, and London: Duke University Press, 1990), p. 126.

12 George Oppen, 'Myth of the Blaze', *New Collected Poems* (New York: New Directions, 2002; Manchester: Carcanet Press, 2003), p. 247.

13 The account that follows is drawn from David McAleavey, 'Oppen: His Impact' in *The Oppens Remembered*, pp. 149–59.

14 George Oppen, 'Route', *New Collected Poems*, p. 196.

15 George Oppen, '"Meaning Is to Be Here": A Selection from the Daybook', *Conjunctions:10* (Spring 1987), edited by Bradford Morrow, p. 199.

16 Edgar Jones, 'Shell shocked', *Monitor on Psychology*, American Psychological Association, Vol. 43, No. 6 (June 2012); see <http://www.apa.org/monitor/2012/06/shell-shocked.aspx>

17 For further information about the legacy of the First World War, see Shephard, *A War of Nerves: Soldiers and Psychiatrists 1914–1994*.

18 Liana Chase began her research looking at the resilience of

Bhutanese refugees in both the US and Nepal. See, for example, '"Solving Tension": coping among Bhutanese refugees in Nepal', *International Journal of Migration, Health and Social Care*, Vol. 9, Issue 2 (2013), pp. 71–83 and also '"In our community, a friend is a psychologist": An ethnographic study of informal care in two Bhutanese refugee communities', *Transcultural Psychiatry*, Vol. 54, Issue 3 (May 2017), pp. 400–422. She is now completing her PhD at SOAS, University of London, in 'Ecologies of mental health care in post-earthquake Nepal survivors'.

19 'Life contains an inescapable element of actual suffering . . . at the very least we will suffer illness, old age and death'. Chris Pauling, *Introducing Buddhism* (Cambridge: Windhorse Publications, 1990), p. 46.

20 For more information on the 'heart-mind', see Liana's article, 'Making Peace in the Heart-Mind: Towards an ethnopsychology of resilience among Bhutanese refugees', *European Bulletin of Himalayan Research*, Vol. 43 (2013), pp. 144–66.

21 See also Brandon A. Kohrt's 'Nepali concepts of psychological trauma: the role of idioms of distress, ethnophyschology and ethno-physiology in alleviating suffering and preventing stigma', *Culture, Medicine and Psychiatry*, Vol. 34 (2) (2010), pp. 322–52. See <https://www.ncbi.nlm.nih.gov/pmc/articles/PMC3819627/>

22 Useful background on the war, and its legacy, can be found in Prashant Jha's *Battles of the New Republic: A Contemporary History of Nepal* (London: C. Hurst & Co., 2014).

23 For more information on TPO Nepal, see <http://tponepal.org/>

24 According to some research, the levels of PTSD were as low as 5.2 per cent: N. P. Luite et al., 'Mental health problems in the aftermath of earthquakes in Nepal', *European Psychiatry*, Vol. 33 (March 2016), pp. 194–5. See <https://www.europsy-journal.com/article/S0924-9338(16)00357-6/abstract>

25 For details of this study, and some background on Narrative Exposure Therapy, see Arun Jha and Suraj Shakya, 'Rationale for conducting PTSD Research and Challenges of Recruiting and Training Volunteers to Screen and Treat PTSD among the Nepal 2015 Earthquake Survivors', *Nepal Medical Association*, Vol. 53, Issue 199 (July–September 2015), pp. 202–7. See <https://pdfs. semanticscholar.org/cd39/f948f31554720f85f2a05032a1e876f99a43. pdf > and also Arun Jha and Suraj Shakya,'Identification and treatment of Nepal 2015 earthquake survivors with post-traumatic stress disorder by non-specialist volunteers', *Indian Journal of Psychiatry*, Vol. 59, Issue 3 (2017), pp. 320–27. See <https://www. ncbi.nlm.nih.gov/pmc/articles/PMC5659082/>

26 For more on NET, see 'Narrative Exposure Therapy', published by the American Psychological Association, July 2017. See <http:// www.apa.org/ptsd-guideline/treatments/narrative-exposure-therapy. aspx>

27 Bessel van der Kolk, *The Body Keeps the Score: Mind, Brain and Body in the Transformation of Trauma* (London: Allen Lane, 2014), p. 42.

28 See, for example, Neeraj Chauhan,'Nepal girls trafficked into India up by 500% in last 5 years: SSB report', *The Times of India*, 31 March 2018. See <https://timesofindia.indiatimes.com/india/ nepal-girls-trafficked-into-india-up-by-500-in-last-5-years-ssb- report/articleshow/63551720.cms>

29 The ideas that follow about trauma and its treatment are indebted to Bessel van der Kolk's excellent book, *The Body Keeps the Score*. Some of his opinions are summarised in this interview: <https:// www.psychotherapy.net/interview/bessel-van-der-kolk-trauma>. 'From my vantage point as a researcher we know that the impact of trauma is upon the survival or animal part of the brain. That means that our automatic danger signals are disturbed, and we

become hyper- or hypo-active: aroused or numbed out. We become like frightened animals. We cannot reason ourselves out of being frightened or upset', p. 1; accessed May 2018.

30 Interestingly, given so many of the people I have spoken to have suffered afflictions of the throat, Nancy had had a tonsillectomy when she was a child, and had been held down during the procedure. She remembered struggling and trying to get away. Levine suggests that this process of shaking and running from the tiger allowed Nancy to finally make her escape. See interview, Victor Yalom and Marie-Hélène Yalom, 'Peter Levine on Somatic Experiencing', Psychotherapy.net, April 2010; <https://www.psychotherapy.net/interview/interview-peter-levine> and also P. Levine, *Waking the Tiger: Healing Trauma* (Berkeley, CA: North Atlantic Books, 1997).

31 For more information on Lisa's work in Nepal, please see her website 'Lion Path' at <http://www.lionpath.org/current-operations/>

32 As Peter Levine explains in his interview 'Peter Levine on Somatic Experiencing', 'one of the things that Bessel van der Kolk showed when he first started to do trauma research with functional MRIs is that when people are in the trauma state, they actually shut down the frontal parts of their brain and particularly the area on the left cortex called Broca's area, which is responsible for speech. When the person is in the traumatic state, those brain regions are literally shut down, they're taken offline.' See <https://www.psychotherapy.net/interview/interview-peter-levine>

PART FOUR: SILENCE

1 George Oppen, 'One must not come to feel that he has a thousand threads in his hands, / He must somehow see the one thing; / This is the level of art / There are other levels / But there is no other level of art', 'Of Being Numerous', section 27, *New Collected Poems*

(New York: New Directions, 2002; Manchester: Carcanet Press, 2003), p. 180.

2 Joan Didion, *The Year of Magical Thinking* (London: Fourth Estate, 2005).

3 Robert Kirk, *Walker Between Worlds: A New Edition of the Secret Commonwealth of Elves, Fauns and Fairies*, edited by R. J. Stewart (Shaftesbury, Dorset: Element Books, 1990).

4 See Peter Levine in interview, Victor Yalom and Marie-Hélène Yalom, 'Peter Levine on Somatic Experiencing', Psychotherapy. net, April 2010 at <https://www.psychotherapy.net/interview/ interview-peter-levine> and also Jane Compson, who has discussed the fact that, unlike in Somatic Experiencing, in meditation practitioners are not able to 'titrate' their experience, which can lead to distress: Jane Compson, 'Meditation, Trauma and Suffering in Silence: raising questions about how meditation is taught and practiced in Western contexts in light of a contemporary trauma resiliency model', *Contemporary Buddhism*, Vol. 15, Issue 2 (2014), pp. 274–97.

5 Sara Maitland, *A Book of Silence* (London: Granta, 2008), p. 78.

6 Marina Abramovic is an artist who famously performed the show *The Artist Is Present* at New York's Museum of Modern Art in 2010, where she sat in silence in the gallery for over 736 hours in total, while members of the public queued to sit opposite her.

7 The details of this experiment are outlined in Daniel Gross's article, 'This Is Your Brain on Silence', *Nautilus*, Issue 16 (21 August 2014). See <http://nautil.us/issue/16/nothingness/this-is-your- brain-on-silence>

8 See, for example, '50,000 heart deaths a year caused by traffic noise', Transport & Environment, 28 February 2008. See <https:// www.transportenvironment.org/press/50000-heart-deaths-year- caused-traffic-noise>

9   The details of this experiment are outlined in Daniel Gross's article, 'This Is Your Brain on Silence', *Nautilus*, Issue 16 (21 August 2014). See <http://nautil.us/issue/16/nothingness/this-is-your-brain-on-silence>

10 Geoffrey Durham, *Being a Quaker: A guide for newcomers*, 1st edn (London: Quaker Quest, 2011) is an excellent introduction to Quaker beliefs and practices, including their use of silence.

11 L. Bernardi et al., 'Cardiovascular, cerebrovascular, and respiratory changes induced by different types of music in musicians and non-musicians: the importance of silence', *Heart*, Vol. 92, Issue 4 (April 2006), pp. 445–52.

12 See, for example, Sadat Malik, 'Silence, Please: The regenerative effects of peace and quiet', *The Practice*, 28 July 2016. See <http://thepracticelondon.org/mindfulness/silence-please-the-regenerative-effects-of-peace-and-quiet/>

13 'Finnish silence can be golden, says American expert', Uutiset website, 18 January 2013. See <https://yle.fi/uutiset/osasto/news/finnish_silence_can_be_golden_says_american_expert/6454371>

14 Karin Paish, 'How I quit talking for 6 months', *The Mirror*, 5 August 1999; The Free Library, 1999 MGN LTD, 2 August 2018. See <https://www.thefreelibrary.com/How+I+quit+talking+for+6+months.-a060440416>

15 'Words cannot be wholly transparent. And that is the "heartlessness" of words', George Oppen, 'Route', *New Collected Poems*, p. 194.

16 Maitland, *A Book of Silence*, pp. 108–14.

17 A useful history of the convent and Tyburn Tree are given on the convent's website. See <https://www.tyburnconvent.org.uk/tyburn-tree>

18 The documentary *Tyburn Convent – Gloria Deo* gives a good sense of the lives of the Tyburn sisters. See <https://www.tyburnconvent.org.uk/site.php?menuaccess=157>

19 A useful history of the Triratna movement can be found in Vajragupta's *The Triratna Story* (Cambridge: Windhorse Publications, 1995).

20 Miguel Farias and Catherine Wikholm's *The Buddha Pill* (London: Watkins Publishing, 2015) gives a timely exploration of the current vogue for mindfulness, and asks if meditation can actually change you.

21 See Farias and Wikholm, *The Buddha Pill*.

22 Daniel Ingram explains the Arising and Passing Away, and other stages of consciousness, in depth in his book *Mastering the Core Teachings of the Buddha: An Unusually Hardcore Dharma Book* (London: Aeon Books, 2008).

23 'The Dark Side of Meditation', Round Table interview hosted by Emily Horn, Buddhist Geeks, 20 June 2014. See <https://www.youtube.com/watch?v=kTLr0gqQTuU>; accessed March 2018.

PART FIVE: LAST WORD

1 Mary Oppen, *Meaning a Life, an Autobiography* (Boston, MA: Black Sparrow Press, 1978), p. 70.

2 George Oppen, 'The Hills', *New Collected Poems* (New York: New Directions, 2002; Manchester: Carcanet Press, 2003), p. 75.

3 *The Selected Letters of George Oppen*, edited by Rachel Blau DuPlessis (Durham, NC, and London: Duke University Press, 1990), p. 349.

4 *The Selected Letters of George Oppen*, p. 319.

5 *The Selected Letters of George Oppen*, p. 286.

6 *The Selected Letters of George Oppen*, p. 310.

7 Rachel Blau DuPlessis, 'Introduction' to *The Selected Letters of George Oppen*, p. 346. She describes the letters as 'Trying to sort out their feelings of love, confusion and pain at Oppen's worsening condition.'

8 George Oppen was diagnosed with Alzheimer's in 1982 and died on 7 July 1984.

9   'George Oppen interviewed by L. S. Dembo, Madison, Wisconsin, April 25, 1968', *Speaking with George Oppen: Interviews with the Poet and Mary Oppen, 1968–1987*, edited by Richard Swigg (Jefferson, NC, and London: McFarland and Company, 2012), p. 20.

10 George Oppen, 'Two Romance Poems', *New Collected Poems*, p. 261.

BIBLIOGRAPHY

Andrews, Sophie, *Scarred* (London: Hodder & Stoughton, 2007)

Andrews, Sophie, 'The Interview', BBC World Service, 7 March 2010. See <https://www.bbc.co.uk/programmes/p006g30n>; accessed January 2018

Bernardi, L. et al., 'Cardiovascular, cerebrovascular, and respiratory changes induced by different types of music in musicians and non-musicians: the importance of silence', *Heart*, Vol. 92, Issue 4 (2006), pp. 445–52

Bowlby, Rachel, 'Introduction', Sigmund Freud and Josef Breuer, *Studies in Hysteria*, translated by Nicola Luckhurst (London: Penguin, 2004)

Bullard, D., 'Bessel Van Der Kolk on Trauma Development and Healing', Psychotherapy.net. See <https://www.psychotherapy.net/interview/bessel-van-der-kolk-trauma>; accessed May 2018

Butler, Pat (dir.), *Chad Varah: The Good Samaritan*, Torchwood Production, Channel Four, 9 August 1992

Chase, L., 'Making Peace in the Heart-Mind: Towards an

ethnopsychology of resilience among Bhutanese refugees', *European Bulletin of Himalayan Research*, Vol. 43 (2013), pp. 144–66

Chase, L., '"Solving Tension": coping among Bhutanese refugees in Nepal", *International Journal of Migration, Health and Social Care*, Vol. 9, Issue 2 (2013), pp. 71–83

Chase, L., '"In our community, a friend is a psychologist": An ethnographic study of informal care in two Bhutanese refugee communities', *Transcultural Psychiatry*, Vol. 54, Issue 3 (May 2017), pp. 400–422

Chauhan, Neeraj, 'Nepal girls trafficked into India up by 500% in last 5 years: SSB report', *The Times of India*, 31 March 2018. See <https://timesofindia.indiatimes.com/india/nepal-girls-trafficked-into-india-up-by-500-in-last-5-years-ssb-report/articleshow/63551720.cms>

Cline, Tony, 'Selective Mutism in Children, Changing Perspectives Over Half a Century', in Benita Rae Smith and Alice Sluckin (eds), *Tackling Selective Mutism* (London: Jessica Kingsley Publishers, 2014)

Compson, J., 'Meditation, Trauma and Suffering in Silence: raising questions about how meditation is taught and practiced in Western contexts in light of a contemporary trauma resiliency model', *Contemporary Buddhism*, Vol. 15, Issue 2 (2014), pp. 274–97

Cope, Stephen, 'Introduction', George Oppen, *Selected Prose, Daybooks, and Papers* (Oakland, CA: University of California Press, 2007)

Davidson, Michael, 'Distant Life', *The Oppens Remembered:*

Poetry, Politics, and Friendship, edited by Rachel Blau DuPlessis (Albuquerque: University of New Mexico Press, 2015)

Davidson, Michael, 'Introduction', George Oppen, *New Collected Poems* (New York: New Directions, 2002; Manchester: Carcanet Press, 2003)

Didion, Joan, *The Year of Magical Thinking* (London: Fourth Estate, 2005)

Dillon, Niamh, 'Interview with Chad Varah', *National Life Stories: Pioneers in Charity and Social Welfare* series, audio recordings, 2004-12-09 & 2005-01-05. Accessed at British Library Sound Archive

Dubuc, Bruno, 'The Amgydala and Its Allies', *The Brain* (2002), Canadian Institutes of Health Research. See <http://thebrain.mcgill.ca/flash/a/a_04/a_04_cr/a_04_cr_peu/a_04_cr_peu.html>; accessed June 2016

DuPlessis, Rachel Blau, 'Introduction', *The Selected Letters of George Oppen*, edited by Rachel Blau DuPlessis (Durham, NC, and London: Duke University Press, 1990)

Durham, Geoffrey, *Being a Quaker: A Guide for Newcomers* (London: Quaker Quest, 2011)

Ensler, Eve, *Insecure at Last: Losing It in Our Security-obsessed World* (New York: Villard Books, 2006)

Ensler, Eve, *In the Body of the World* (London: Virago Press, 2013)

Ensler, Eve, 'How We Made: The Vagina Monologues', *The Guardian*, 4 February 2013

Ensler, Eve, 'The Power of Story' podcast (Sydney Opera House, 12 December 2017). See <https://www.sydneyoperahouse.

com/backstage/podcasts/its-a-long-story/eve-ensler.html>; accessed January 2018

Ensler, Eve, 'Hair', *The Vagina Monologues, 20th Anniversary Edition* (London: Virago Press, 2018)

Ensler, Eve, 'Introduction to the 20th Anniversary Edition', *The Vagina Monologues, 20th Anniversary Edition* (London: Virago Press, 2018), pp. xv–xvi

Farias, Miguel and Catherine Wikholm, *The Buddha Pill: Can Meditation Change You?* (London: Watkins Publishing, 2015)

'Finnish silence can be golden, says American expert', Uutiset website, 18 January 2013. See <https://yle.fi/uutiset/osasto/news/finnish_silence_can_be_golden_says_american_expert/6454371>

Freud, Sigmund and Josef Breuer, *Studies in Hysteria*, translated by Nicola Luckhurst (London, Penguin, 2004)

George, Rose, 'Blood Speaks', *Mosaic*, 11 March 2014. See <https://mosaicscience.com/story/menstrual-taboo-periods-shame-women/>

Gross, Daniel, 'This Is Your Brain on Silence', *Nautilus*, Issue 16 (21 August 2014). See <http://nautil.us/issue/16/nothingness/this-is-your-brain-on-silence>

Hatlen, Burton, 'Introduction', *George Oppen, Man and Poet*, edited by Burton Hatlen (University of Maine: National Poetry Foundation, 1981)

Hatlen, Burton and Tom Mandel, 'Poetry and Politics: A conversation with George and Mary Oppen', in *George Oppen, Man and Poet*, edited by Burton Hatlen (University of Maine: National Poetry Foundation, 1981)

'Hoohaa in US over Monologues play', BBC News website, 9 February 2007

Hustvedt, Asti, *Medical Muses: Hysteria in Nineteenth Century Paris* (New York: W. W. Norton & Co.; London: Bloomsbury, 2011)

Hurst, A., *Medical Diseases of War* (London: Edward Arnold, 1918)

Ingram, Daniel, *Mastering the Core Teachings of the Buddha: An Unusually Hardcore Dharma Book* (London: Aeon Books, 2008)

Jha, A. and Shakya, S., 'Rationale for conducting PTSD Research and Challenges of Recruiting and Training Volunteers to Screen and Treat PTSD among the Nepal 2015 Earthquake Survivors', *Nepal Medical Association*, Vol. 53, Issue 199 (July–September, 2015). See <https://pdfs.semanticscholar.org/cd39/f948f31554720f85f2a05032a1e876f99a43.pdf>

Jha, A. and Shakya, S., 'Identification and treatment of Nepal 2015 earthquake survivors with post-traumatic stress disorder by non-specialist volunteers', *Indian Journal of Psychiatry*, Vol. 59, Issue 3 (2017), pp. 320–27. See <https://www.ncbi.nlm.nih.gov/pmc/articles/PMC5659082/>

Jha, Prashant, *Battles of the New Republic: A Contemporary History of Nepal* (London: C. Hurst & Co, 2014)

Johnson, Maggie and Alison Wintgens, *The Selective Mutism Resource Manual* (Abingdon: Routledge, 2001)

Johnson, Maggie and Alison Wintgens, *Can I tell you about Selective Mutism? A Guide for Family and Friends* (London: Jessica Kingsley Publishers, 2012)

Jones, Edgar, 'War Neuroses and Arthur Hurst: a pioneering medical film about the treatment of psychiatric battle casualties', *Journal of the History of Medicine and Allied Sciences*, Vol. 67, Issue 3 (May 2011). See <https://www.kcl.ac.uk/kcmhr/publications/assetfiles/historical/jones2011-warneuroses.pdf>

Jones, Edgar, 'Shell Shocked', *Monitor on Psychology*, American Psychological Association, Vol. 43, No. 6 (June 2012). See <http://www.apa.org/monitor/2012/06/shell-shocked.aspx>

Jones, Edgar and Simon Wessely, *Shell Shock and PTSD: Military Psychiatry from 1900 to the Gulf War* (New York and Hove, Sussex: Psychology Press, 2005)

Jones, Edgar and Simon Wessely, 'Battle for the Mind: World War 1 and the birth of military psychiatry', *The Lancet*, 8 November 2014. See <https://www.kcl.ac.uk/kcmhr/publications/assetfiles/2014/Jones2014e.pdf>

Karki, C., 'Suicide: Leading Cause of Death among Women in Nepal', *Kathmandu University Medical Journal*, Vol. 9: 3, Issue 35 (July–September 2011)

Kibble, David G., *The Samaritans*, Religious and Moral Education Charity series (Oxford: Pergamon Press, 1983)

Kirk, R., *Walker Between Worlds: A New Edition of the Secret Commonwealth of Elves, Fauns and Fairies*, edited by R. J. Stewart (Shaftesbury, Dorset: Element Books, 1990)

Kohlmeier, Jonathan, *Learning to Play the Game: My Journey Through Silence* (Morrisville, NC: Lulu Publishing Services, 2016)

Kohrt, Brandon A., 'Nepali concepts of psychological trauma: the role of idioms of distress, ethnopsychology and ethnophysiology in alleviating suffering and preventing stigma', *Culture Medicine and Psychiatry*, Vol. 34 (2) (2010), pp. 322–52. See <https://www.ncbi.nlm.nih.gov/pmc/articles/PMC3819627/>

Kolk, Bessel van der *The Body Keeps the Score: Mind, Brain and Body in the Transformation of Trauma* (London: Allen Lane, 2014)

Langton, James, 'Stars come out for V-Day', *Daily Telegraph*, 14 February 1998

Levine, P., *Waking the Tiger: Healing Trauma* (Berkeley, CA: North Atlantic Books, 1997)

Looff, David, *Appalachia's Children: The Challenge of Mental Health* (Lexington, KY: University of Kentucky Press, 1971)

Luite, N. P., 'Mental health problems in the aftermath of earthquakes in Nepal', *European Psychiatry*, Vol. 33 (March 2015), pp. 194–5. See <https://www.europsy-journal.com/article/S0924-9338(16)00357-6/abstract>

MacCaig, Norman, 'Aunt Julia', *The Many Days: Selected Poems of Norman MacCaig* (Edinburgh: Polygon, 2010)

Maitland, Sara, *A Book of Silence* (London: Granta, 2008)

Malik, Sadat, 'Silence, Please: The regenerative effects of peace and quiet', *The Practice*, 28 July 2016. See <http://thepractice london.org/mindfulness/silence-please-the-regenerative-effects-of-peace-and-quiet/>

Marahatta, K. et al., 'Suicide burden and prevention in Nepal: the need for a national strategy', *WHO South East Asia Journal of Public Health*, 6:1 (April 2017)

McAleavey, D., 'Oppen: His Impact', *The Oppens Remembered: Poetry, Politics, and Friendship*, edited by Rachel Blau DuPlessis (Albuquerque: University of New Mexico Press, 2015)

McDougall, W., *An Outline of Abnormal Psychology* (London: Methuen & Co., 1926)

Myers, C. S., 'A contribution to the study of shell shock', *The Lancet*, 13 February 1915, p. 316. See <http://jmvh.org/wp-content/uploads/2012/12/A-Contribution-to-the-Study-of-Shellshock.pdf>

'Narrative Exposure Therapy', American Psychological Association, July 2017. See <http://www.apa.org/ptsd-guideline/treatments/narrative-exposure-therapy.aspx>

'Nepal: two years on, the government continues to fail marginalised earthquake survivors', Amnesty International, 25 April 2017. See <https://www.amnesty.org/en/latest/news/2017/04/nepal-two-years-on-the-government-continues-to-fail-marginalised-earthquake-survivors/>

NHS, 'Selective Mutism', August 2014. See <http://www.nhs.uk/conditions/selective-mutism>; accessed August 2016

Nicholls, Peter, *George Oppen and the Fate of Modernism* (Oxford: Oxford University Press, 2007)

'Objectivist', in 'Glossary of Poetic Terms'. See <http://www.poetryfoundation.org>; accessed 10 May 2018

Oppen, George, 'The Mind's Own Place' from *Selected Poems* (New York: New Directions, 1962). See at <http://www.poetryfoundation.org/articles/69407/the-minds-own-place>; accessed May 2018

Oppen, George, '"Meaning Is to Be Here": A Selection from the Daybook', *Conjunctions:10* (Spring 1987), edited by Bradford Morrow

Oppen, George, *The Selected Letters of George Oppen*, edited by

Rachel Blau DuPlessis (Durham, NC, and London: Duke University Press, 1990)

Oppen, George, *New Collected Poems* (New York: New Directions, 2002; Manchester: Carcanet Press, 2003)

Oppen, Linda, 'Turquoise', *The Oppens Remembered: Poetry, Politics, and Friendship*, edited by Rachel Blau DuPlessis (Albuquerque: University of New Mexico Press, 2015)

Oppen, Mary, *Meaning a Life, an Autobiography* (Boston, MA: Black Sparrow Press, 1978)

Oppen, Mary, and Dennis Young, 'Conversation with Mary Oppen', *The Iowa Review*, Vol. 8, Issue 3 (Fall 1988), pp. 18–47. See <https://doi.org/10.17077/0021-065X.3657>

Paish, Karen, 'How I quit talking for 6 months', *The Mirror*, 5 August 1999; The Free Library, 1999 MGN LTD, 2 August 2018. See <https://www.thefreelibrary.com/How+I+quit+talking+for+6+months.-a060440416>

Pauling, Chris, *Introducing Buddhism* (Cambridge: Windhorse Publications, 1990)

Pound, Ezra, 'Preface to *Discrete Series*', George Oppen, *New Collected Poems* (New York: New Directions, 2002; Manchester: Carcanet Press, 2003)

Rigby, Jennifer, 'Nepal earthquake anniversary: one year on, not one home rebuilt by government', *Daily Telegraph*, 25 April 2016. See <https://www.telegraph.co.uk/news/2016/04/25/nepal-earthquake-anniversary-one-year-on-not-one-home-rebuilt-by/>

Roberts, F. J., 'Clinical Theology: An Assessment', *Theological Students Fellowship (TSF) Bulletin*, Vol. 64 (Autumn 1972), pp. 21–5

'Sex and the Citizen', *Picture Post*, 15 September 1951. See *Picture Post* Historical Archive; accessed 2 August 2018

Shephard, B., *A War of Nerves: Soldiers and Psychiatrists 1914–1994* (London: Jonathan Cape, 2000)

Smith, Benita Rae, and Alice Sluckin, 'Introducing Selective Mutism and an Overview of Approaches', in Benita Rae Smith and Alice Sluckin (eds), *Tackling Selective Mutism* (London: Jessica Kingsley Publishers, 2015)

Solomon, Andrew, *The Noonday Demon: An Atlas of Depression* (New York: Scribner; London: Chatto & Windus, 2001; revised edn, 2014)

Spasaro, Sheila A. and Charles E. Shaefer (eds), *Refusal to Speak: Treatment of Selective Mutism in Children* (Lanham, MD: Rowman & Littlefield, 1999)

'Suicide Leading Cause of Death in Men aged 20–49 in England & Wales', Campaign Against Living Miserably (CALM), 18 February 2014. See <https://www.thecalmzone.net/2014/02/onssuicidereport/>; accessed January 2018

Sutton, Carl, 'An Experiential Introduction to Selective Mutism', in Carl Sutton and Cheryl Forrester (eds), *Selected Mutism in Our Own Words, Experiences in Childhood and Adulthood* (London: Jessica Kingsley Publishers, 2015)

Swan, Susan Celia and Purva Panday Cullman, 'Say It, Stage it, V-Day at Twenty', *The Vagina Monologues, 20th Anniversary Edition* (London: Virago Press, 2018; originally published 1998)

Swigg, Richard (ed.), *Speaking with George Oppen: Interviews with the Poet and Mary Oppen, 1968–1987* (Jefferson, NC and London: McFarland and Company, 2012)

'The Dark Side of Meditation', Round Table interview by Emily Horn, Buddhist Geeks, 20 June 2014. See <https://www.youtube.com/watch?v=kTLr0gqQTuU>; accessed March 2018

Vajragupta, *The Triratna Story* (Cambridge: Windhorse Publications, 1995)

Varah, Chad, 'A Parson Puts His Case', *Picture Post*, 10 November 1951. See *Picture Post Historical Archive* online; accessed 2 August 2018

Varah, Chad, *Before I Die Again* (London: Constable, 1992)

Wallace, Marjorie, *The Silent Twins* (London: Vintage, 1998)

Yalom, Victor and Marie-Hélène Yalom, 'Peter Levine on Somatic Experiencing', interview, Psychotherapy.net, April 2010. See <https://www.psychotherapy.net/interview/interview-peter-levine>

Zimet, Julian, 'Notes from Memoirs and Conversations of Julian Zimet', *The Oppens Remembered: Poetry, Politics, and Friendship*, edited by Rachel Blau DuPlessis (Albuquerque: University of New Mexico Press, 2015)

SELECTED ADDITIONAL RESOURCES

'About Us', Selective Mutism Information & Research Association (SMIRA). See <http://www.smira.org.uk; accessed February 2016

Clarke, J. W., 'A Gift of Bricks: Silence and the Poetry of George Oppen', *PN Review*, No. 185 (2009), pp. 33–7

Cline, Tony and Sylvia Baldwin, *Selective Mutism in Children*,

2nd edn (London and Philadelphia: Whurr Publishers, 2004; first published 1994)

De-la-Noy, Michael, *Acting as Friends: The Story of the Samaritans* (London: Constable, 1987)

Hoffman, Eric R., *Oppen: A Narrative* (Bristol: Shearsman Books, 2013)

Jenkins, G. Matthew, 'Saying Obligation: George Oppen's Poetry and Levinasian Ethics', *Journal of American Studies*, Vol. 37, No. 3 (December 2003), pp. 407–33

Kabat-Zinn, Jon, *Full Catastrophe Living: How to cope with stress, pain and illness using mindfulness meditation*, revised edn (London: Piatkus, 2013; originally published 1990)

Kimmelman, B., 'George Oppen's Silence and the Role of Uncertainty in Post-War American Avant-Garde Poetry', *Mosaic: a journal for the comparative study of literature*, Vol. 36, Issue 2 (June 2003), pp. 145–62

Lebrun, Yvan, *Mutism* (London: Whurr Publishers, 1990)

Peel, Barnaby (dir.), *My Child Won't Speak*, Landmark Films, BBC One, 2 February 2010

Sutton, Carl, *Selective Mutism in Adults: An exploratory study* (MSc Dissertation, University of Chester); available at <http://www.ispeak.org.uk>; accessed June 2016

Tramer, M., 'Electiver Mutismus bei Kindern', *Zeitschrift für Kinderpsychiatrie*, Vol. 1 (1934), pp. 30–35, translated by Anja Boeing

PERMISSIONS CREDITS

ACKNOWLEDGEMENTS

I OWE A HUGE DEBT of gratitude to everyone who took the time to speak to me during my research and whose stories helped to shape this book. Thank you.

I am also incredibly thankful to my family, for their unwavering support, not just in the writing of this book, but in everything, and for their willingness for our intertwined stories to find their way into the world.

I am grateful to the Society of Authors, for their generous work in progress grant, which allowed me to complete this book – and to my agent Kirsty McLachlan at David Godwin Associates, who first noticed the potential in a slightly incoherent idea about silence.

Thanks also to the whole team at Canongate for their unfailing support and for guiding me through this process, and particularly to my editor Jo Dingley for her patience and insight, and for knowing what it would take to make this work.

And finally, I want to thank Christa, for her endless tolerance, and for always listening. I love you.

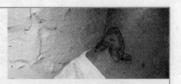

Shortlisted for the
Baillie Gifford Prize
for Non-Fiction 2018

Thomas Page McBee

Amateur

A reckoning with gender, identity and masculinity

'Blazingly wise'
A L Kennedy

'Essential'
Deborah Levy

'Absolutely fascinating'
Nikesh Shukla

'Superb'
Attitude Magazine

'Eye-opening'
Guardian

'A heck of a tale'
Financial Times

'Radical'
Observer

'As much a reconciliation
as an emancipation'
Sunday Times

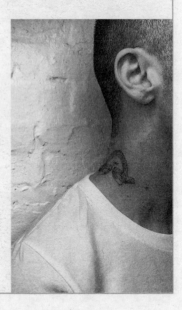

'Brave, honest and touchingly human'
Guardian

CANON GATE

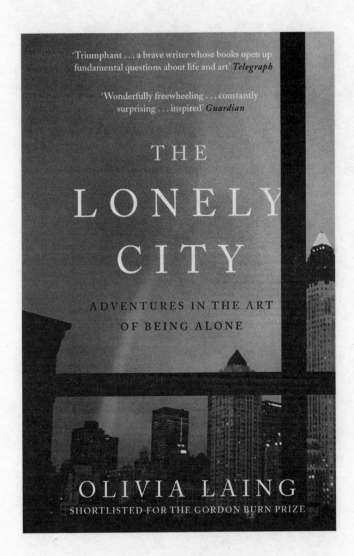

'Triumphant . . . a brave writer whose books open up
fundamental questions about life and art' *Telegraph*

'Wonderfully freewheeling . . . constantly
surprising . . . inspired' *Guardian*

THE
LONELY
CITY

ADVENTURES IN THE ART
OF BEING ALONE

OLIVIA LAING

SHORTLISTED FOR THE GORDON BURN PRIZE

'A fierce and essential work'
Helen Macdonald

CANON▌▌GATE

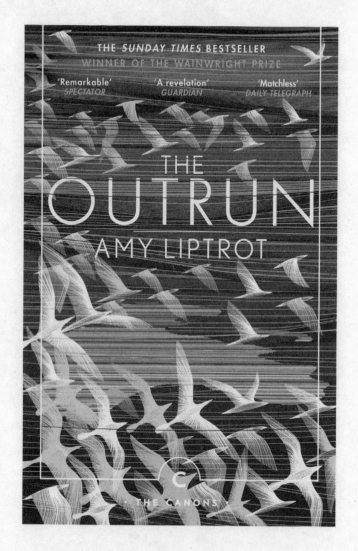

THE *SUNDAY TIMES* BESTSELLER
WINNER OF THE WAINWRIGHT PRIZE

'Remarkable'   'A revelation'   'Matchless'
SPECTATOR   GUARDIAN   DAILY TELEGRAPH

THE
OUTRUN

AMY LIPTROT

THE CANONS

'A luminous, life-affirming book'
Olivia Laing

CANON ‖ GATE